D0832178

WEIGHT LOSS SURGERY
DOES NOT TREAT
FOOD ADDICTION

CONNIE STAPLETON, PH.D.

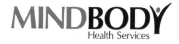

MINDBODY
Health Services

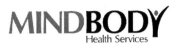

Copyright © 2017 Connie Stapleton, Ph.D.

Published by Mind Body Health Services, Inc.

All rights reserved.
No part of this book may be reproduced, stored in a retrieval system, or
transmitted by any means, electronic, mechanical, photocopying, recording,
or otherwise, except for brief passages in connection with a review, without
written permission from the author.

ISBN: 978-1548460464

DEDICATION

This book is for those many patients whose food addiction was ignored by bariatric professionals unwilling to acknowledge, or give direction for, the treatment of food addiction. Food addiction is a disease similar to obesity in that it affects millions, is disregarded by many professionals as well as lay persons, and carries a great deal of stigma. Like obesity, addiction is a disease and must be treated as such. Treating the disease of obesity does not treat the disease of addiction; each disease must be treated separately. May all patients who are being treated by bariatric professionals soon be screened for food addiction. If a patient meets the criteria for food addiction, may the bariatric professional assist them in finding the treatment they need to address their disease of addiction.

ACKNOWLEDGEMENTS

First and foremost, I thank every person who opts to read this book! I appreciate your willingness to learn more about food addiction and how to treat it.

I have tremendous gratitude to those people who struggle with obesity and/or food addiction, who have shared with me stories of their lives, their difficulties and their successes. I hope this book represents you honestly and with the compassion I feel for the diseases you fight on a daily basis.

For those who volunteered to read and edit this book, I thank you over and over. Special thanks go out to Paulene Relkey, Amy Helms, Lynn Murray, Katy Merriman, Carla Halkias, and Cheryl Grimes Quade. Your insights and suggestions were extremely helpful!

Andrea and David Schroeder. I consider you both to be very instrumental in my development as a professional. Your support of my work has helped me in ways I could never express. Thank you for being friends, both personally and professionally.

Reeger Cortell, you are a wonderful inspiration to me. I admire your professionalism, your curiosity and the essence of who you are. Thank you for being part of my professional journey. And thank you for your amazing podcast, the Weight Loss Surgery Podcast with Reeger Cortell on iTunes.

Personally, my love and thanks go to my three very best friends of many decades. Diane Hay, Diane Shanafelt and Sally Buras, you are my go-to friends for all of my life "stuff." Thank you for loving me at my best and my worst and always encouraging me to follow my passion and my dreams. My world is whole because I have you as my girlfriends. You're everything the Lovebug cannot be!

Two people without whom I could not manage my job, who also did very thorough editing are Kelsey Potthast and Emily Ellis. My right and left hands! You two are amazing, willing to drop other projects and focus on whatever is at hand, and always do an exceptional job! Kelsey, thank you for running my life and making it seamless for me. I appreciate you, both personally and professionally beyond measure. Emily, we need you more than you can imagine! Thank you for being so very professional, so dedicated and so compassionate.

Steven Little, I can always count on you to make my work look amazing. You are a remarkably talented man and always come through for me. You're a pretty amazing human being as well, and have my utmost respect all the way around.

My Lizzy, you are encouraging and beyond hard-working. Thank you for sharing kind words and always supporting the team and me in our endeavors.

There is not enough thanks or gratitude for my Lovebug. You are unending in your support of me, the work I do, and the work we do together. Without you, there would not be such an amazing big picture, either in our work lives, or in our personal lives. You make it happen. Thank you for sharing every aspect of your life with me.

And thank you to "my babies." Always and forever you bring me joy.

TABLE OF CONTENTS

PREFACE

I have worked in the field of addiction and Recovery for the past 25 years. My work in the last 15 years has primarily been in the arena of bariatric medicine, with a specific focus on bariatric surgery, or "weight loss surgery."

Weight regain is a tremendous concern for many patients who opt to have bariatric surgery. This concern is valid, as a large number of patients do regain some to most to all of the weight they lose in the first couple of years following their surgical procedure.

Due to my background in addiction, it didn't take long while working in bariatrics before I realized that the percentage of patients we treat who regain a substantial amount of weight in the years following surgery, do so in relation to a disease they battle. A disease in addition to the disease of obesity: food addiction.

Food addiction is a controversial topic among medical and psychological specialists. However, many patients earnestly identify themselves as being addicted to food. It is my sincere belief that by not addressing the issue of food addiction with our patients, and failing to provide them with guidance for getting help to treat their food addiction, we are being unethical and "doing harm" to our patients. This book is intended to educate both patients and bariatric professionals about the disease of food addiction.

Please note that I intentionally capitalized the "R" in Recovery throughout the book. Recovery is, to me, a sacred process deserving of being capitalized to express it as such. Recovery is a healing process, not just meant to physically relieve the intense cravings for, and the illogical, sometimes extreme behaviors associated with food and eating. Recovery is a deeply personal, internal, often spiritual process of letting go of the need for control, allowing permission to experience human feelings, learning to accept and deal with life as it is, and developing a healthy relationship with self. The results of the Recovery process include re-establishing a healthy relationship with food and often improving interpersonal relationships with others.

Here's to your Recovery! Enjoy the journey.

CHAPTER ONE

THE M.D. AND THE PH.D. SQUARE OFF

The room was already packed. People were standing along the sides of, and against the walls. It was a typical hotel conference room, divided in half by a basketball court sized movable partition on one side and a darkly painted wall on the other. The lighting was dim and the temperature too cold, as is often the case in conference rooms. Three panelists were scheduled, but I was the only one currently seated at the table in front of the room. The other two speakers slowly worked their way to the front, stopping to chat with meeting attendees along the way. We had plenty of time before the session began, so no one was in a hurry.

The moderator for the panel was a bariatric surgeon. I hadn't ever met him, but I already felt fairly comfortable with him. I had recently listened to an episode of the Weight Loss Surgery Podcast on which he had been the interviewee. The woman who created the podcast, Reeger Cortell, is a friend of mine. She and I had recently shared a lively discussion after I listened to the hour-long interview with Dr. Surgeon. I processed my thoughts about this man's attitude and practices related to bariatric surgery with my friend.

"Wow! He's got quite a distinct perspective, given he's a surgeon," I shared. I was driving back from Atlanta to my home in Augusta while she and I chatted. I often use those two hours and 40 minutes (but who's timing?) to listen to podcasts. When I have decent reception, which isn't as often as it should be given the current calendar year, I catch up on the phone with my friends. My phone-chatting time in life is limited, given my days are spent in sessions with patients. The evenings fly by while I catch up on paperwork, exercise, write and snuggle with my husband, "the Lovebug." Weekends are spent enjoying pure baby bliss: changing diapers, wiping runny noses, attempting to feed toddlers who are much less interested in food than in my cell phone, playing chase and "Red Light, Green Light," reading classic children's books, getting as many sloppy kisses and hugs as I can, and falling asleep waiting for the babies to fall asleep. Grandchildren – they truly are God's reward in life!

Reeger, who created the *Weight Loss Surgery Podcast*, works by day as a Nurse Practitioner in a bariatric clinic. She agreed with my assessment of Dr. Surgeon. "He definitely approaches his patients differently than many bariatric surgeons."

I added, "I especially like that he has a whole-person perspective about bariatric surgery. He understands the importance of positive self-talk, maintaining an optimistic attitude, and realizing that there is much more to bariatric surgery than a given procedure on a specific day." We continued to address the many helpful points made by this young surgeon who shared a great deal of his personal journey on the podcast. "As a psychologist, I appreciate that he's been through some struggles of his own and has learned a great deal about himself. He shared those aspects of his journey and applied many of the concepts he learned along the way with his patients. I found myself agreeing almost wholeheartedly with what he shared. Except for one thing," I offered.

"I think I can guess what that one area of disagreement was," Reeger mused.

My mind rushed back to the scene at hand. The man who had been the topic of my conversation with Reeger sat down next to me at the table in front of the still-gathering crowd. The noise level was high. Well over one hundred people chatted amongst themselves. Much laughter emanated from the crowd of patients and professionals meeting or reuniting after months since they last saw one another.

"Doctor," I extended my hand to shake his. "You may not recall my name. I'm Connie Stapleton. I recently sent you a message on your Facebook page after I listened to your podcast interview with Reeger."

"Oh, yes," he responded. His eyes had that look indicating he was searching the files of his brain, trying to recall a message from me and attempting to recall my name.

I saved him from having to come up with something on the spot. "That was a very refreshing perspective you shared. Not many surgeons appear to appreciate as fully as you the fact that bariatric surgery affects every area of a person's life. You noted the internal and interpersonal changes that accompany the process associated with surgery." That statement sparked a congenial, albeit very short conversation about the information he shared on the podcast.

"There was one thing about which I disagreed with you," I noted.

"That being?" he inquired.

"I've worked for 25 years in the addiction field as a certified addictions counselor. For the past twelve years, I have worked specifically in the bariatric community. I firmly believe that for some people, eating and food are addictions," I shared without apology.

"Well," he quipped, "You're only as good as your training. OB/GYN's think they're surgeons, too." He stood up and walked to the speaker's podium as the other two panelists took their seats.

"OB/GYNs *do* perform surgeries," I said aloud. To myself, I fumed, "Did he really just say that? How insulting! How arrogant!" It was a good thing I wasn't the first presenter, whose talk went off without a hitch. Admittedly, I didn't actually hear much of that presentation due to the storm of thoughts and emotions swirling through my mind.

I couldn't help remembering the time years ago when my twin daughters were on a local recreation-league basketball team. They were ten years old. The volunteer coach was the father of one of the other kids on the team. He was giving up his time to help all of our kids. That's a sacrifice in this busy world. It was a sacrifice I genuinely appreciated, being the mother of three kids myself as well as a full-time PhD student, juggling classes, internships and research projects. Volunteer coaching, something my husband did every season as well, is truly an act of love and dedication.

After one particular game, during which the Dad Coach had been more animated than usual, I approached him. It had been obvious to me over the past few weeks that Dad Coach may have forgotten that these children were ten years old, hardly old enough to be competing for a position in the major leagues. They weren't even trying out for the high school varsity team. In fact, these girls weren't trying out for anything. They were playing on a city rec team, mostly for fun, since the majority of them weren't very good yet. Clumsy little legs flailing about, tears sprung loose over a skinned knee on the court, and still the occasional throwing of the ball in the direction of the other team's goal. Dad Coach had, now and then, gotten excited and his voice rose a bit. Not a big deal. However, last week and this week in particular, he must have been getting worried about the team record or something. His comments and voice tone were no longer appropriate for ten year-old-children, regardless of gender.

I about came down from the bleachers after the game. A few minutes earlier, he bellowed to one of the girls (not even my child), "What the hell are you doing out there?" Mind you, I have a potty mouth from hell, so his bellowing of the H-E-double-toothpicks didn't faze me. It was the anger and the intensity with which he screamed that inflamed me.

"Excuse me, Dad Coach," I said after we, yes, won the game. (Okay, I didn't call him Dad Coach). I smiled. "I wanted to let you know how much I appreciate all the time you give up to spend with our girls, scheduling practices and being at all of the games." He beamed. I glared. "I also want you to know how much I do NOT appreciate the volume and tone with which you chastise these TEN-YEAR-OLD CHILDREN." He stared, stunned. I walked away.

I wanted to give Dr. Surgeon a piece of my mind right there in front of the room filled with people, like I had the Dad Coach that day. I did not appreciate the way he had spoken to me, nor did I appreciate how he had negated my training in addictions or the surgical training of OB/GYNs.

My mind focused as I heard Dr. Surgeon announce, "Our next speaker is a licensed psychologist who has, I have just learned, worked in the field of addictions for twenty years and in bariatrics for the last ten. Let's welcome licensed psychologist, Dr. Connie Stapleton." Polite applause.

As I stood up, Doctor Surgeon said, "Before I hand over the podium, how many of you, if you're a patient, consider yourself to be a food addict?" Nearly every hand in the room shot up. He sat down. I then shared with the audience, verbatim, in a falsely playful tone, the conversation he and I had minutes earlier, before the session began. *"So there, you arrogant SOB,"* I gloated internally. I ended my pre-speech speech by saying, "And let me tell you why I believe that some people who struggle with losing weight and keeping it off have an addiction to food/eating. When someone knows they have problems in their life that are caused by, or worsened by their use of a substance or behavior – in this case, the problems being excess weight and comorbid health problems and the substance being food – and the person wants to stop using that substance or wants to stop that behavior … BUT THEY CANNOT DO SO… we're talking about an addiction. If you don't like the word addiction, simplify the matter. If something causes problems in your life, it's a problem."

I went on from there to discuss the topic I had been assigned for this particular breakout session. My concluding statements were as follows: "I began this afternoon talking about food being an addiction for some people. Let me end today by saying, *Weight Loss Surgery does NOT Treat Food Addiction.*" Loud applause erupted.

CHAPTER TWO

WELL, DAMN!

"Listen, Dr. Stapleton," Cheryl began as we sat together in my therapy office, which patients tell me daily is "cozy." The warm light from the several (six) floor lamps barely provides enough light in the windowless room to see well. I can't stand the overhead, oh-so-bright-and-obnoxious fluorescent lighting of the medical-exam-room-turned-therapy-office that would accost patients if I didn't have the half dozen lamps. Fluorescent lighting is not conducive to delving into personal, intimate issues in therapy.

Secretly, every time a patient tells me how "cozy" my office is, I want to shout, "COZY?!!! It's COZY if you're in here for an *hour*. The room has NO windows. The horribly dim lighting causes my eyes to play tricks on me all day long. The four tan walls close in on me more every hour, and the gray and brown furniture does NOTHING to brighten the place. The rocking chair, although amazingly awesome and super comfy just PUTS ME TO SLEEP. I need to be fully present during my time with you. This room is not COZY for six or eight or ten hours at a time. It's a PRISON! I'm an outdoor kind of gal and I'm losing my mind in here!" But I say, as much for the patient's sake as for my own

PMA (positive mental attitude), "It is cozy. Very cozy." (For the record, in case you're wondering why I don't just change it, it's because I can't. I rent this room at the bariatric practice and the owner prefers all of the décor in the building to match. I completely understand and respect this. I just don't like it!)

Enough about my issues…

Cheryl sat on the firm gray sofa. There was one oversized feather-stuffed pillow behind her back for support and another held tightly across her abdomen, a hallmark of many a patient trying to conceal their weight. "When I had the Lap Band surgery six years ago, I figured I wouldn't be able to overeat ever again and wouldn't have to worry about regaining weight yet another time."

"How did you regain the 70 pounds you lost after your procedure?" I asked in a non-judgmental, inquisitive tone.

"I kept those 70 pounds off for almost two years," Cheryl remarked sullenly, as she sat with her eyes fixed on the floor, deep in thought. After a few minutes of silence as her thoughts gelled, I gently asked, "And then what happened?"

Without lifting her head or her eyes, as tears spilled down her face and onto her magenta and navy patterned blouse, she nearly whispered, "The same thing that's happened a hundred times in the past. I gave in to old habits and lost the battle. Again."

The Battle.

Yep. You, like Cheryl, may have fought that battle with weight:

- *after you had your babies*
- *since you were a baby*
- *following steroid treatment that lasted a year*
- *from the minute you hit puberty and every day thereafter*
- *since your divorce was final*
- *beginning the day you moved out of your parents' home*
- *following that miserable hysterectomy*
- *after you put on "the college freshman 15"*
- *beginning in mid-life*
- *since FOREVER!*

What a battle it's been – in many a literal sense. The definition of battle as a *noun*, according to Dictionary.com is, "a fight; any conflict or struggle." As a *verb*, battle means, "to work very hard or struggle; strive." You've literally had to *fight* and *struggle* in relation to your weight for some, most, or all of your life.

You've been *fighting* with your body all these many years, *striving* to lose weight, participating in this diet or that diet or the other diet, none of the diets "working." In spite of your efforts to count calories, count carbs, count sugar grams, or count steps, your body would only cooperate in losing "a few pounds." Even if you lost a lot of pounds, they always found their way back to your belly, your thighs, your face, or your arms.

As part of the battle with weight you *fought* to maintain your dignity in society. Sadly, in spite of all the obesity awareness and education, people continue to judge, blame, shame, punish, abuse, and humiliate other human beings who struggle with this stubborn disease.

Perhaps you've *battled* a family member or two who insist you're "lazy," and that is why you haven't been able to lose weight "on your own" (as in, without surgery). Or maybe a spouse or parent *fought against you* by sabotaging your efforts those times you did lose weight.

"After my weight loss surgery, my spouse kept bringing home foods like snack cakes, licorice, coffee drinks filled with sugary syrups, and peanut butter candy… all of my favorite unhealthy foods! We argued about it constantly. I told him I didn't want him to bring those things into the house but in he'd saunter from work, announcing on the way through the door that he had brought me a 'surprise.' He was the one who got the surprise when I finally took the dessert he brought and shoved it down the sink, turning on the garbage disposal before taking even one bite. He eventually told me he was afraid that I would leave him because I lost so much weight. My feeling so much better about myself was a threat to him. I assured him I loved him no matter what I weigh – just as he has always loved me, regardless of what I weighed. We were able to talk through our feelings, even though it wasn't easy. I asked him to be supportive of my journey – and he has been ever since. I have made more of an effort to let him know how much he means to me, too!" Men and women regularly tell me versions of this scenario. Sadly, this picture doesn't always end well. The divorce rate for couples following weight loss surgery is far higher than the national average.

Have you, as a person struggling with obesity, had to *fight* to obtain or maintain employment? Has it been a struggle to get a job in a society where weight is erroneously equated with ineptitude? Keith, weighing in at 320 pounds, recently told me, through tears he worked hard to abate, about his humiliation, anger and shame when, at a recent job interview, he was told he didn't get the job because he was "a health insurance risk." To add insult to injury, the hiring committee added, "We're also concerned about the image you would project to our congregation." Keith was interviewing for the position as pastor of a prominent church. "I met all of the credentials and had paid my dues pastoring for years in smaller communities. My heart yearns to serve as pastor of a larger church, where I can grow and learn and in turn, positively affect the lives of others."

Have you been overlooked for promotions within your company and suspected it was related to your weight? Ron, a very tall, very intelligent engineer, shared that he had put in for "promotion after promotion" within his organization for a period of three years, to no avail. Since losing 135 pounds after weight loss surgery, he has experienced an equal number of promotions in an even shorter period of time. He also asked for a raise. He said he would never have had the confidence to do this before losing weight. Much to Ron's joyous surprise, he was granted the increase in pay.

Indeed, your struggle with weight has been a battle. Those stubborn pounds seem to stalk you when you manage to shed them from your physique. You have fought and fought, sometimes with temporary "success," but inevitably followed by the storming of the food troops, leading to regaining those 20, 30, or 70 pounds, *"plus some."* The battles along the way… from the days of tormenting classmates and critical coaches, through years of dealing with the cruelty of siblings, to the well-intentioned efforts at "help" by stymied parents and extended family members, and on into the adult world of judgmental bosses, coworkers, peer groups, and society in general, are so exhausting!

No fight, however, has been as brutal as the war you've been waging with *yourself* in the weight loss battle that has become your life. *What?* There's no use denying this. I've heard it from too many people over too many years for it not to be true. You brutally batter yourself with negative self-talk. STINKIN' THINKIN'. For more than a few folks, it turns out that STINKIN' THINKIN' can be a subconscious way of setting oneself up for further punishment via food. For example:

- "I don't know why I even bother," a sentiment often followed by "giving in" to decadent carbs that ease the emotional pain of yet another dieting defeat.

- "I hate the way I look and feel" is soothed by the sweet salve of cookies, ice cream, and melt-in-your-mouth milk chocolate.
- "I've tried everything I can imagine and nothing works for me," a sorrowful statement of defeat, soon drowned by the richness of butter cream icing on raspberry lemon cheesecake.

*Oh, **that** kind of self-talk.* Yes, that. It's stinkin' thinkin' and it often leads the way to the vicious merry-go-round of the abuse cycle between self and food. Stinkin' thinkin' is present where addiction lives.

THE WAY YOU TALK TO YOURSELF, ABOUT YOURSELF, IS A POWERFUL CONTRIBUTING FACTOR TO THE REASONS YOU HAVEN'T BEEN ABLE TO SUSTAIN WEIGHT LOSS IN THE PAST. STINKIN' THINKIN' IS COMMONPLACE WHEN ADDICTION IS PRESENT.

Why would anyone engage in such a personal cycle of abuse with words and with food?

Read the following examples and note the stinkin' thinkin' embedded in these real-life scenarios. Consider how these comments intensify low self-esteem, reinforce low self-efficacy (one's belief in their ability to succeed), and increase self-doubt.

- Megan lost 40 pounds in four months using a prepackaged meal diet program. We explored the reasons she decided to "quit" this diet program. "**I messed up again** when I chose that diet. **Another one of my brilliant ideas, I guess.** I wanted to lose weight so badly. **As usual, I wasn't thinking clearly** or I would have realized I couldn't live on pre-packaged meals forever. I had to stop socializing with my friends because going out to eat is what we do. I got lonely. So, **of course**, as soon as I started hanging out with my friends and quit the diet, I regained all 40 of those pounds in no time. **My mom was right. I guess I *am* a slow learner.**"
- Susan lost 86 pounds in 15 months following a strict low-carb diet. It took her 6 short months to regain every pound. As we talked about what led her to re-invite her "true love," bread, back into her life, she said, "I didn't like the kind of attention I was getting from men at the lower weight. **I'm not physically attractive**, so I figured they were paying attention to me so they could get what they really wanted from me. **What did I expect?**

I didn't want *that* kind of attention so I decided to eat what I like and **not have to worry about more rejection** when I told people I wouldn't sleep with them."

- Martin, after losing 65 pounds by cutting out sodas and putting the kibosh on his nightly routine of devouring two bowls of cereal before bed, started to feel proud of himself. His father, who had always been critical of him, unexpectedly stopped by Martin's house one evening, a very rare occurrence. Martin was hoping his father would have something positive to say about his weight loss. Instead, the words that fell out of his father's mouth were, "Who the hell are you trying to impress? You're still the same underachiever you've always been." Martin said to me, **"I knew he was right. I'm not a 'reach for the stars' kinda guy, so why bother with all the hard work it takes to lose a few lousy pounds?"**

It's not hard to hear the negative self-talk in these examples. However, Megan, Susan and Martin don't recognize it in themselves. Even when I pointed out to them the ways they were speaking negatively about themselves, they were surprised and struggled to hear the ways in which they were belittling themselves.

Like them, you are probably unaware of the ways you speak negatively to yourself, about yourself. It takes quite a bit of self-awareness, along with feedback from trusted friends, for us to hear it. When a person begins to hear their own versions of stinkin' thinkin', they can then begin the task of making the connection between that form of self-abuse (the negative self-talk) and the subsequent negative behavior. They can also then make positive changes. These types of positive changes are part of Recovery from addiction, which you will read much more about in later chapters.

NEGATIVE SELF-TALK (AS WELL AS NEGATIVE SELF-THOUGHTS AND NEGATIVE SELF-IMAGE) ARE DIRECTLY RELATED TO NEGATIVE, SELF-SABOTAGING BEHAVIOR. PEOPLE IN THE THROES OF ADDICTIONS SELF-SABOTAGE IN A NUMBER OF WAYS.

Sometimes, the negative messages about self are much less overt than in the above examples. In some cases, it's not so obvious that a person thinks poorly of himself, but their behavior represents it. For example, Michele is a single mother of four. Michele's ailing father lives with her and the children. "Finding time for myself **just isn't gonna happen.**"

Ellen is the soccer mom, the self-appointed office social chair, and the extended family "go-to gal." She explained, "The whole extended family depends on me. I am the one they call when there's a crisis or a decision to be made. I'm the one they ask for advice. I'm the one who is supposed to have all the answers for everybody about everything. **How could I possibly** take time to cook healthy meals, let alone get to the gym?"

Naomi explained how she takes care of **"everyone but myself."** I hear this so often that I think someone needs to make it into a song that tells the real story. The lyrics might go something like this (hum to the tune of Twinkle Twinkle Little Star):

> I take care of my kids and mom,
> My husband and his brother Tom,
> There's no time to care for me
> I don't matter, don't you see?
> To hide the way I really feel,
> I eat in secret … that's how I deal.

Women like Michele and Ellen and Naomi (and yes, many men, as well) are genuinely and legitimately very busy as a result of the demands we all face in this too-busy world. The unspoken and underlying message is, "**I don't matter** in comparison to others." I've heard that world-renowned people, famous for helping scores of others in this world, are diligent about taking time to care for themselves (physically, mentally, and spiritually) so they have the strength they need to care for others. We could all stand to remember the importance of this wisdom.

Obviously, there are stages in our lives when we have less time for a full regimen of self-care than at other times. However, rare is the season of life we cannot care adequately for both ourselves and others. Parents: do you want to teach your children that it's good to give all of yourself to the care of others at the detriment of your own health? I think not… yet, so many people rationalize their lack of self-love and self-care with this martyr-ish attitude of "caring for everyone but myself." (Yes, I said martyr. If you're offended, keep reading to the end of this book. Being a martyr is a coping mechanism. I'm not judging. You'll understand ...).

A negative self-image, which is expressed through harsh words about oneself (i.e., negative self talk, or stinkin' thinkin'), is often an underlying reason people don't follow through with good self-care.

NEGATIVE SELF-ESTEEM SILENTLY, AND OFTEN SUBCONSCIOUSLY, "DRIVES THE BUS" THAT LEADS PEOPLE BACK TO UNHEALTHY EATING HABITS, A LACK OF ADEQUATE EXERCISE, AND TO THE EMOTIONAL COMFORT THAT FOOD PROVIDES THEM.

Yes, I am saying that people often regain their weight because they feel icky about themselves. They say rude things to and about themselves, and think horrible things about themselves. No, it's not the *thinking* that causes weight gain. It's the eating of unhealthy food to soothe the harsh self-talk and self-battering that results in weight regain. And the eating may be about food addiction.

NEGATIVE THOUGHTS LEAD TO NEGATIVE FEELINGS. NEGATIVE THOUGHTS AND NEGATIVE FEELINGS LEAD TO NEGATIVE BEHAVIORS. NEGATIVE THOUGHTS, NEGATIVE FEELINGS, AND NEGATIVE BEHAVIORS ARE ALL-TOO-COMMONLY PRESENT WHEN ONE IS ACTIVE IN AN ADDICTION.

To be sure, we will return to this topic throughout the book... because as it turns out, self-talk, self-thoughts, self-image, self-esteem... will be key players in this food addiction thing!

WHAT I THINK ABOUT WEIGHT LOSS SURGERY

I am a big fan of weight loss surgery. I support weight loss surgery for the following reasons:

- Research tells us that only 1 person out of 100 who have at least 100 pounds to lose will do so and keep it off without weight loss surgery.

- Weight loss surgery results in the loss of approximately 60% of a person's excess weight in a relatively short amount of time.

- Bariatric surgery leads to improvements in health (oftentimes significant improvements) and gives the person a greater opportunity to keep the excess weight off for life.

Here's the catch. Sadly, I don't believe patients are very well educated about the realities of life following weight loss surgery. I know patients are not very often educated about food addiction prior to having bariatric surgery. Food addiction needs to be treated as a separate disease from obesity. To make matters even more complicated, I'm not sure it's even possible to adequately prepare anyone for the realities of life after bariatric surgery. Similarly, it's difficult to get a person to understand they may have an addiction when they are only interested in getting their excess weight off as quickly as possible. In their minds, weight loss surgery is the complete answer.

Have you ever been married? In my video series, MindPrep, designed for use in weight loss surgery programs to help prepare patients more fully for surgery and life after surgery, I talk about how preparing for weight loss surgery is like preparing for a wedding. Here's part of the script from the first MindPrep video:

"I'm going to tell you a story and want you to picture it as clearly as possible as I describe the scenario. Ready? Let's start…

Imagine a starry-eyed young couple, madly in love, who have made the decision to get married. They become engaged and begin making their plans to live happily ever after. Most of their friends and relatives are thrilled for them. They offer congratulations, support, encouragement and help in planning the wedding. Others are, whether openly or in private, questioning the decision of this young couple to take the plunge into matrimony. They wonder whether they are "ready," speculating that perhaps they are too young, or aren't really aware of what they are getting into.

The young couple?! They aren't paying attention to any negativity. Of course they're aware of the statistics on divorce! Ah, but they are in love, and intend to stay that way forever! Sure - they understand there will be "rough patches" in marriage. But they are certain they will sail right through any murky waters and get back on track in no time. They plan to talk through any and all issues that arise. They have even attended their three marriage preparation classes and are ready to get this show on the road. After all, there's a wedding to plan!

Well… those of us who have been married a decade or two sit back and smile knowingly at young couples such as this. We were in their shoes once upon a time, fully believing we would breeze through any tough spots encountered on the meandering roads of marriage. Some things we skated through with ease. At other times, we likely wondered how we would survive! One thing is for certain. People who have been married for any length of time know that the "easy" times ebb and flow, but every day of a healthy marriage requires effort.

There *is* a relevant point in all this marriage talk. A few years back, all three of my children got married within a ten-month period of time. Needless to say, we were very wedding-focused during those months! It occurred to me as we went through the process of our children's weddings that the surgical weight loss journey and marriage have a lot in common!

Back to our smitten couple... Leading up to a marriage proposal, the lovebirds talk and daydream for hours on end. They are giddy that they have finally found one another and grateful that their turn has finally arrived. The one they have waited for their whole life has been delivered! Married life will be all they ever dreamed of and they can finally see the path to HAPPILY EVERY AFTER! The first step, of course, is the engagement.

That alone presents a number of questions:

- Is the timing right?
- Where should I pop the question?
- Is the ring just right?
- Then there's the QUESTION: WILL YOU MARRY ME?
- Oh my goodness... What will The ANSWER be?!

HMMM... How about the person who is considering weight loss surgery? They ponder and daydream about what weight loss surgery could mean for them and how they would look and feel after losing their excess weight. Perhaps they have waited years or even a lifetime to find a real option to losing that excess weight! And now, finally – the opportunity has arrived. This means their dreams can finally come true. *They* can actually see a light to *their* HAPPILY EVER AFTER!

Like a marriage proposal, there are similar questions related to the PROPOSED surgical procedure:

- Is the timing right?
- Do I have insurance coverage?

- Do I have enough information?
- How do I know this will work?
- The big QUESTION: Should I or shouldn't I?
- And then – there is The ANSWER!

For both the wedding and the surgery there comes a decision:

- We will get married!
- I *will* have weight loss surgery!

The minute a love-struck young couple is formally betrothed, the wedding planning begins. The list of decisions to make is mind-boggling:

- In what month should we get married?
- Where will we have the wedding?
- How about the reception? Where do we want that?
- How many attendants will we have?
- What sort of flowers will we have?
- What music do we want?
- Who will officiate?
- Who will we invite?
- How much is this going to cost?
- The DETAILS seem endless: blood tests, a marriage license, bridesmaid gifts, flower choices, menu options, music arrangements…
- Oh – and do we HAVE to go to the marriage classes? After all, things are so great with us. Sure – maybe half of marriages fail, but that won't be us… we are going to do this right!

Like our couple, eager to get married, once a person has definitively made the decision to have weight loss surgery, the attention turns to the details:

- When should I plan to have the surgery?
- What hospital will I go to?
- Who will my surgeon be?

- What type of surgery should I have?
- Who will my support people be?
- Who should I invite on my journey?
- How much is this going to cost?
- The DETAILS seem endless: there's the endoscopy, the sleep study, blood tests, and EKG, the nutritional evaluation, the psychological evaluation...
- Oh – and MUST I go to the nutrition classes and have a psychological evaluation before I have my surgery? I know that lots of people have weight loss surgery and gain their weight back, but I'm different! I know what I'm doing and I WILL do this right!

Engaged couples and people preparing for weight loss surgery go through periods of intense enthusiasm and also some DOUBT during the period of time leading up to the big event:

- Perhaps family members don't react with the level of enthusiasm or support they expected.
- The betrothed and the surgical candidate may have unwanted questions pop up in their minds... questions like:
  - What if I'm not quite ready?
  - What if something goes wrong?
  - What if, what if, what if...????

"Normal" doubts make an appearance in the process of preparing for a wedding or for weight loss surgery. In spite of these doubts, people most often come to the conclusion: I'm ready. I'm prepared. I know this is what I want to do and I KNOW I will be successful!

ONWARD AND FORWARD!

People who have decided to have weight loss surgery usually do have some doubts and fears. However, by the time they've gotten to the point that they need surgery, possibly due to having numerous health comorbidities, people are often desperate to get the weight off. Surgery seems like "The Answer!" The vast majority of patients (I did NOT say '*all patients*,' so please don't get upset if this doesn't pertain to you) painstakingly check off the list of requirements they must meet in order for their insurance and/or bariatric center to approve them for surgery. Some complain about it every single step along the way. Most people don't have the chutzpa (the audacity) to say out loud what is written all over their faces, (although some do): "*I just want the damn surgery already! WHY must I jump through all of these hoops?*"

Just this morning, I informed a 28-year-young woman that she needed some additional education prior to being approved for surgery. She is young, which means she has a lifetime to enjoy the benefits of weight loss. Because she is young, this also means if she regains the weight because she wasn't prepared for surgery, she may regret having had it in the first place. I shared with her that the purpose of requiring additional steps prior to being approved for bariatric surgery were to help her make necessary changes in her food choices prior to having surgery and to give her a preview of what she would need to do after surgery. I offered her several options of ways to obtain the information she needed, and provided different choices for proving she was willing to put forth the effort required of her following surgery. All options required ten weeks of effort prior to being re-evaluated for readiness. She haughtily replied, "Then I don't think I'll have the surgery at all." She got up and walked out of the office. Apparently those ten weeks to help establish good habits were going to require too much of her.

DO YOU KNOW WHAT THE MOTTO OF AN ADDICT IS?
"I WANT WHAT I WANT WHEN I WANT IT."

The Hoops. Why the Hoops?

The literal answer to the question, "*WHY must I jump through all of these hoops?*" is, "We want you to be as prepared as possible for life after weight loss surgery so you are able to have improved health and to maintain a healthy weight for the rest of your life." I know, just a few paragraphs ago, I said it's not really possible to be prepared for life after weight loss surgery. Well, it's not possible to know what childbirth is like before you go through it either, but lots of people go to all sorts of classes to prepare for that, as well.

Those of us ushering you through the dreaded hoops required for weight loss surgery preparation and insurance approval are hoping to give you a realistic idea of what to expect after you leave the hospital.

Once you are back at home with your fresh surgery wounds and your small stomach pouch, you no longer have the physical ability to "abuse" food for the moment.

Hear me when I say that prior to surgery, the medical team is working hard in an attempt to prepare patients for knowing how to live a healthy life using the tool that bariatric surgery provides. Too often, patients don't really care about being properly "prepared." They just want to get to the O.R. (operating room) and get this weight loss thing happening already! Being unprepared and uninformed are additional causes leading to the frequency of weight regain. To make matter worse, current preparation by the medical professionals, as we have discussed, rarely includes educating patients about food addiction. The blind leading the blind here. I say this because most medical professionals don't understand food addiction, which makes it unlikely they'll be teaching the patients about it.

And that is where my work comes in.

HOW I GOT INVOLVED

I started working in the field of weight loss surgery many years after I began my professional work as a psychologist. I was working as the staff psychologist at a medical college, seeing medical and dental and nursing students for therapy. I was also working part time in private practice when my professional shift into the weight loss surgery world occurred. I received a form letter in the mail, which had been canvased to all of the psychologists in the area. It was sent by a company looking to hire a licensed psychologist who had previous experience in both sales and addiction. I knew I had the job.

It wasn't arrogance. I simply knew the chances of many other licensed psychologists having specific work experience in both sales and addiction was unlikely. Before I went back to school to get my Master's degree and my PhD, I had worked in direct sales. This is going to give you a clue about how old I really am… I sold World Book Encyclopedias… DOOR TO DOOR! Can you even imagine doing such a thing in this day and age? First of all – are you even old enough to know what a set of encyclopedias is?! Secondly, can you just see me – this young college graduate with three little ones at home in diapers, out in the world with my little sales kit, canvassing the neighborhood (or rural Iowa farm land) looking for swing sets, toys strewn around the yard, and other signs of homes where children lived? Into those yards I strode, ready to educate…

I continue to educate all these years later, although to a much different population. My work with bariatric patients began in 2004. Why was that company who sent the letter seeking a psychologist with prior sales and addiction experience? Because this company knew what they were doing. They knew that a high percentage of people opting for weight loss surgery **a)** may have come from a home where one or both parents was an addict of some sort, and **b)** may have an addiction of their own (to food, alcohol, drugs, etc.). This company understood that it was the time spent with patients both before and after surgery that would prepare them for long-term success in maintaining a healthy weight for life. The company wanted to hire a psychologist who could "sell" patients on the idea of participating in pre- and post-operative education related to bariatric surgery. They also wanted a psychologist who had experience working in addictions because the hiring company knew many people seeking bariatric surgery have food addictions.

This company offered a thorough pre- and post-surgical psycho-educational program for patients pursuing weight loss surgery. Patients were required to attend a minimum of ten topical sessions prior to being approved for surgery. The topics weren't even related to the surgical procedure itself. They were much more important! Patients were taught how to deal with family issues, problems with friends, marital difficulties, self-esteem, grief over losing one's friend, "food," and other issues related to the emotional aspects of how life and relationships change after surgery. They were also taught about food addiction. It was made clear to patients that if they suffered from food addiction, they would need to treat the food addiction separately from their obesity! Weight loss surgery would not, and will not, treat food addiction, whether the addiction is physiological or psychological in nature.

The topics of the required seminars offered through this program addressed all the areas of a person's life that change after weight loss surgery. The focus was on how to deal effectively in life without using FOOD as a means of escape or avoidance. If people are not given replacement "tools" to use when they are stressed, they are likely to return to the tool that helped them in the past. In this case, the tool prior to surgery was food. In cases of physiological addiction, patients were informed of the need to abstain from all trigger foods/substances. The pre-surgical classes did what all good therapy does:

taught people healthy ways to deal with life's ups and downs. Food is meant to be an enjoyable way to provide our bodies with the nutrition needed to carry us through life. Food is not meant to help a person avoid anger, obscure sadness, squelch loneliness or allay boredom.

The patients associated with this program were also offered ongoing weekly classes following surgery. A year's worth of weekly topics were offered, but the patients were welcome to attend the sessions for as many years as they wanted at no additional charge. The post-op classes focused on various aspects of living life fully after weight loss and learning how to deal with the many changes in one's life.

The emphasis on "aftercare," the education following a treatment or procedure, is widely utilized by addiction treatment programs. Program directors at addiction treatment facilities understand the need for solid support and ongoing education after a person stops "using" a substance or behavior in an addictive manner, or as a way to avoid experiencing feelings and/or the realities of life. That is why, in this case, the employer seeking a psychologist was looking for a person with experience in both addiction and sales. They knew a psychologist with this education and experience could develop a comprehensive program for pre- and post- surgical patients.

Having sales experience was also helpful because there was a "program fee" to cover the cost of hiring a psychologist to provide these classes all year long! The sales training proved helpful in "convincing" patients that the pre- and post-op education was essential for their long-term welfare. The psychologist had to "sell" them on the benefits of the cost for the program.

When I knocked on doors selling children's books, it was because I believed in the educational value of World Book Encyclopedias. This made them very easy for me to sell. I also knew, personally and professionally, the value of long-term follow-up support and education following a "treatment." In this case, "treatment" is the surgical weight loss procedure.

The people behind this long-term educational program for surgical weight loss patients, in my opinion, were brilliant and had it right! If all programs offered and *required* this type of preparation prior to surgery and the long-term AFTER-CARE, I believe that many more post-ops would keep their weight off for the long haul.

So why DON'T programs require these types of pre- and post-op psycho-educational classes? Very simply, as more and more medical facilities began offering bariatric surgery and competing for business, patients began to "shop around" for the program where they could have the surgery the quickest. In other words, the fewer "hoops" to jump through, the better – from the eager patient's perspective. That's not a criticism to the patients. I understand that they have lost nearly all hope for losing weight and just want the "magic" of the surgery so they can finally get rid of that excess weight they despise. What they don't understand at a deep, deep level at that point, is that surgery ISN'T MAGIC and does NOT guarantee keeping the weight off. They do not, and cannot, fully understand prior to having weight loss surgery that obesity and weight loss are about more than just pounds and food. Adequate preparation requires more than is currently offered at most programs.

BUT MY PROGRAM IS A CENTER OF EXCELLENCE!

"Well, Dr. Stapleton. That's all interesting information, but I'm not worried. My bariatric center is a Center of Excellence! That's as good as it gets! That means the program *did* provide me with all the preparation that's necessary for surgery."

No. Going to a Center of Excellence simply means you got as much preparation as the medical center is *required to provide*. Which has little to do with receiving a great deal of the information you need to be successful long-term.

If you had your surgery at a "bariatric center of excellence," you *were* as prepared as any patient is going to be, given the current standards. Bariatric programs can earn the designation as a Center of Excellence (COE) by requiring you to see a nutritionist (perhaps for more than one session) and a psychologist or mental health professional. This is typically for one session and often with someone who knows little to nothing about the field of bariatrics or addiction. Patients are also required to attend information sessions with the surgeon and/or other health care professionals to learn about the various surgical procedures. Finally, patients must obtain necessary medical clearances in order to receive their winning lottery ticket, known as **insurance approval**.

Granted, the nutrition information and bits of psychological information is much better than the NO information bariatric patients got prior to surgery in the past. Yet, the information currently provided by Centers of Excellence falls very short of what patients need in order to have an adequate understanding of the numerous contributing factors to obesity, many of which have nothing to do with biology. Neither are patients prepared for the social, emotional and psychological changes they will encounter after the surgery. Marriages change, friendships change, social dynamics change, parent-child relationships change, extended family relationships change and the patient's relationship with him/herself changes. Surgery takes place on one day of a patient's life. The rest of the changes take place after surgery and last for the rest of the patient's life.

Patients are almost certainly NOT informed about food addiction, even if their program is a "Center of Excellence." In fact, it is my belief that few of the professionals working in the Centers of Excellence have even the slightest clue about what food addiction really is.

Centers of Excellence focus on biology, eating better, and exercising more. Behavior modification. Nice information. Necessary information for long term weight management, for sure. Yet, incredibly insufficient information. Most Definitely.

I hate to break it to you, but bariatric programs are a source of big revenue for hospitals. Surgeons make money for themselves and for their hospitals based on the number of surgeries they perform. Trust me when I tell you that the vast majority of surgeons do not care about most of the pre- or post-surgical education of the patient. Very few surgeons give a rat's patootie about the long-term emotional and psychological issues of the patients.

That is NOT to say that there aren't many truly amazing bariatric surgeons and health care professionals who genuinely take care of the patients before, and for many years after the surgery. I have the pleasure of working with several of these amazing men and women.

I know... I know... you LOVE your bariatric surgeon. He/She saved your life! NO THEY DID NOT! YOU made the decision to have weight loss surgery as a step toward improving your health with the hope of lengthening your life and having a better quality of life. YOU are the one who will follow through with healthy eating and exercise, which lead to keeping you healthier. If you are addicted to food, YOU are the one who will get the help you need to treat your addiction. Your surgeon doesn't do any of that. Yes, they are incredibly gifted and talented SURGEONS and I thank God for them! But... please!!!! The surgeon does not get the credit for you changing your life! Nor do you get to blame them if you don't follow through with healthy eating and exercise to keep your weight off. You can't blame anyone if you know you have an addiction to food and don't get help for your addiction.

As wonderful and talented as the surgeons are, I promise you, it isn't going to be the surgeon who teaches you and coaches you and encourages you to make healthy food choices when you're upset or when it's Halloween and candy is everywhere or when it's holiday time and the entire extended family celebrates with a food fest for a solid week. Your mentors and personal support people will be the ones to do that. The ones you can turn to seven days a week, any day of the year. Ultimately, you are responsible for your health and every one of your choices. You alone are responsible for the effort you put into doing whatever is necessary and getting the help you need.

Neither your surgeon nor your Bariatric Center of Excellence (COE) is going to have prepared you to deal with the friends who ditch you because you no longer have anything in common with them. The COEs are not going to help you with your marriage when your partner becomes insecure as your healthy new body struts its stuff like it hasn't since you were 18 years old. No surgeon or other professional at your bariatric center is going to treat a food addiction. That's not their job. Your beloved surgeon isn't going to be there two years after your surgery if you start slipping back into your old habits and begin to panic. They aren't going to wipe your tears if you see the scale inch upward and you are terrified it won't stop. (Yes, there are a few truly amazing surgeons who will do this. A FEW.)

If you have been blessed with a surgeon who offers more than the basics required for Center of Excellence designation, count your blessings. Thank your doctor profusely and frequently. Thank their staff. Refer all of your friends who are considering bariatric surgery to this doctor. Finally, thank yourself, as you are the one who is ultimately responsible for your success.

The Center of Excellence designation is something hospitals seek in order to keep business coming in the doors as much as to ensure patients get good care. Yes, it is definitely in the best interest of the patient to have surgery at a COE, as there are many safeguards put in place designed for the health and safety of the patient. Even the surgeons, most of whom are truly remarkable and do care very much about the short- and long-term wellbeing of the patients, primarily want to get as many people in that operating room as possible. It's how they keep a job – and how they make their own house payments. They are not doing anything bad or irresponsible by wanting to have a lot of business. That IS business! Performing successful surgeries is what these men and women spent many years training to do. In fact, I have to say, having worked at a medical college as the therapist for medical students in training, the public underestimates the sacrifices that medical students make in order to become physicians. In my opinion, no physician should make less than two hundred thousand dollars a year beginning their first day of work after receiving their medical license. Not many people are willing or able to endure the kind of stress these men and women experience as they become physicians.

Surgeons are trained to do surgery. They are not trained to be therapists, nor are they probably interested in that arena. However, a surgeon who is also a good business professional will make sure there are other professionals in place to meet the non-surgical needs of the patients in their bariatric practice.

Good surgeons who are also good business people will put forth the effort and expense to offer additional services within their own practice (such as providing in-house therapists, exercise options such as discounts at local gyms or establishing walking groups as part of the program). Does your surgeon show interest in the long-term emotional changes patients go through? Do they suggest ongoing therapy? Do they warn patients about the risks of alcohol, pain meds and other potential problematic behaviors that can occur after surgery? Do the professionals at your bariatric center educate you about food addiction and provide resources for treatment? Does your bariatric center go above and beyond the educational requirements mandated by political medical organizations? If the answer is yes, your surgeon and their dedicated staff deserve much praise.

Don't believe me? Go get a job at a bariatric center. It won't take you long to learn the cold, hard truth about what I'm saying. Bariatric surgery is a business. The majority of surgeons don't understand the importance of a truly comprehensive program beyond what is required for the almighty Center of Excellence accreditation. Nor are they often willing to invest in the adjunct services to have a thorough program.

And yes, myself and other psychologists who conduct the pre-surgical evaluations are also part of the cold-hearted business world. We make good money doing any sort of psychological evaluation. That is why you need to be extremely careful about the psychologist you choose for your psychological evaluation. Some know little to nothing about weight loss surgery – and don't have any interest in knowing anything about it. They just want the money. *Most* mental health professionals know nothing about food addiction. It's tragic for the patients.

And THAT is why I couldn't NOT.

I COULDN'T NOT

Such proper grammar coming from the PhD… "I couldn't NOT." What exactly couldn't I NOT? I could NOT live with myself if all I did was a one-hour pre-surgical psychological evaluation and think the patient had adequate pre-surgical preparation. And the reason I couldn't live with myself if all I did was a one-hour session is because I know the patients need more. Much more. MUCH MUCH more information about the reality of life after weight loss surgery. And they need to know about food addiction. Because weight loss surgery does not treat food addiction.

How did I know so much about the importance of extensive information and long-term after-care following a treatment procedure? In 1989 I went through an outpatient treatment program for my own addictions to alcohol and prescription pain medication. I learned a lot more in the weekly aftercare sessions following treatment than I did during the six weeks of nightly treatment. In aftercare, I learned about living life fully without the false, short-term "comfort" provided by alcohol, drugs, and other addictive substances and behaviors.

It was in aftercare that I learned how to deal with the issues in my marriage without relying on alcohol or pain medication to calm me down. It was in aftercare that I learned healthy skills for HAVING a healthy marriage. I also learned how to develop healthy friendships, how to improve my self-esteem, how to stop judging myself and others, how to have fun without liquid courage, how to say no and to stand up for myself, how to make decisions, how to address issues with my parents and siblings, and how to be a healthy parent – and to do all of this without my "drug."

My drug of choice was not food (at the time I went to treatment), but I knew enough from my own transferring of addictions (work, male attention, alcohol, pain medications, and exercise) that food, for many bariatric patients, was used for the same reasons I used other substances and unhealthy behaviors: as an attempt to cope with the things in life that I did not know how to deal with in healthy ways. Also, because I had a brain predisposed to addiction.

That is the reason I became involved with bariatric surgery. To me, recovery from a disease is recovery from a disease... whether that disease is alcoholism or obesity or cancer or diabetes or food addiction. There are so many changes in life during and after the "treatment" phase. For those having weight loss surgery, the surgical procedure is their "treatment" option. What most people don't know is that weight loss surgery doesn't treat food addiction. Nor does weight loss surgery treat many of the issues I mentioned having learned about in aftercare. Most people struggling with obesity share many of the same problems of living I had. They need to learn how to cope with the stress and realities of life after surgery without the use of food to provide the "Ahhhh" they are seeking. A bariatric procedure doesn't teach healthy coping skills.

After treatment (for alcohol, drug, or food addiction), people need help learning to live with the many social, physical, emotional and psychological changes in their lives. In addition to educating *patients* on what I know to be essential skills for success following weight loss surgery, which includes teaching about food addiction and recovery, I am also actively "selling," or attempting to educate *health care professionals* about these same things.

The real life information people need to live life fully without their "medication," "drug" or "false sense of comfort" (via alcohol, pills, food, gambling, shopping, etc.) can only be gained by learning healthy coping skills to deal with both physiological cravings for a substance and those emotions, people and situations your "drug of choice" protects you from. In addition, people need constant support from others throughout the recovery process.

You don't really learn how to have a successful marriage until you're living as a married person and struggle through to the other side of some difficult marital issues. You can't really learn to be a successful parent until you've struggled through to the other side of some difficult parenting issues. You can't really learn to be a successful, healthy post-op patient until you've struggled through to the other side of some difficult post-op issues. You can't be successful in recovery from addiction until you know you are an addict and put forth the effort to live in recovery.

You can work through these things on a trial and error basis, always returning to "your old habits" or you can choose to get help from various "lifelines." People can learn healthy tools for working through marital issues, for raising healthy children or for maintaining healthy food habits in many ways: by reading, talking to mentors, attending therapy and/or support groups, watching informative programming or by taking classes. In order to remain in recovery from an addiction, you must opt for abstinence from the addictive substance(s), engage on a regular basis with a solid support network, and learn healthy living skills.

Obviously, the more one can know about how to be successful at something going into it, the better off they'll be. Yet, there are simply some things that we can only fully learn through experience. THAT is why someone who opts to have weight loss surgery needs the most information possible prior to the surgery. It helps to know before surgery what to expect at the time of surgery, and to how to go about living as a successful post-op patient for the rest of their lives.

I am a firm believer in bariatric surgery because it gives people an opportunity for improved health. It literally can save lives. I also believe in weight loss surgery for the potential gifts that have nothing to do with physical health. My passion is about helping people heal the emotional relationship they have with themselves, the most important relationship damaged by an addiction. People who are addicted to food have a damaged relationship with themselves. They carry the burden of shame, negative self-talk, and ongoing self-abuse related to a disease they likely don't understand and definitely don't know how to treat.

When people learn to have a healthy relationship with themselves, they treat their bodies better and heal their unhealthy relationship with food. In the process of healing themselves and treating themselves with more love and respect, they heal other relationships in their lives. Hence, the need for more intensive "pre-surgical hoops" and more post-operative support groups (to include therapy groups and addiction recovery groups). Participation in these groups teaches people how to heal the relationship with themselves.

So now you understand. I could NOT simply conduct a one-hour psychological evaluation for patients hoping to have weight loss surgery and leave it at that. I needed to provide them more information. I needed to give them tools. That is why I created the pre-cursor videos to the current MindPrep video series. I had my son literally video record me in my living room. We recorded several hours of information about maintaining a healthy weight after bariatric surgery. I required all of the pre-op patients to view the videos prior to approving them for surgery because, in all good conscience, I could not rush them through the pre-surgical process without more than a cursory understanding about the surgery and how to live life afterwards. Because guess what?

OBESITY ISN'T JUST ABOUT THE FOOD

Ok. It's a little about the food. Obviously, food has something to do with obesity. Look at this list of common factors contributing to obesity. Please note that "Addiction" is not found on the websites or in articles describing the causes of obesity. I added that to the list myself.

- **Genetics**
- **Culture and Environment**
- **Metabolism**
- **Illness and Medications**
- **Sleep**
- **Personal Behaviors**
- **Psychological Aspects**
- *Addiction*

How often do you see the word FOOD in that list? You don't! Food, for the sake of this discussion, falls into the personal behaviors category. And food is only one aspect of the personal behaviors related to obesity. Food – your personal behaviors with food. What you eat. When you eat. How much you eat. Personal behaviors related to obesity also include exercise. What kind of exercise you do. How often you exercise. Even if you are addicted to food, you are ultimately responsible for what you put in your mouth and whether or not you exercise regularly.

Food is a part of cultures, but only one part of a person's culture and environment. Food may be a large part of a culture or one's home environment, but the bottom line with food, when you're an adult anyway – lies with personal behaviors. *Choices.* You can make changes. It's a choice. Which, of course, I know, is easier said than done, especially if you are a food addict. That's why there are a lot more chapters in the book.

Obviously, there is more to the bigger picture of obesity than what goes into your mouth and how much exercise you get. Otherwise, Personal Choice would be the only thing on the list above. What's important in the realm of getting weight off and keeping weight off is to *focus on the items on the list that you can influence.*

By the way, did they educate you about any of this during your pre-surgical hoop jumping at your Bariatric Center of Excellence? Did your surgeon mention any of this? The psychologist?

PSYCHOLOGICAL ASPECTS OF OBESITY AND ADDICTION

From the list of factors that contribute to excess weight, the most overlooked, and perhaps the most important areas for maintaining a healthy weight are the "Psychological Aspects" and "Addiction." Of course, I'm biased. I'm a psychologist! But let's think through this together. Current protocol for medical and surgical weight loss focus on medical problems related to obesity, nutrition and food consumption, and the "psychological" component under the heading, "behavior modification," which sort of makes me want to cry. Obviously, people need to work on behavior changes (which is code for "eat less and move more"). But for programs to assume food behaviors and exercise alone covers the "psychological" aspects of weight loss is nothing short of absurd. Completely ignoring the issue of addition is blatantly irresponsible! It baffles me, blows my mind, frustrates me, and downright befuddles me that so many smart people can be so damn stupid as to ignore the emotional/psychological/addiction aspects of obesity, weight loss and healthy weight maintenance.

It's all about getting people into the programs (cha-ching, cha-ching), whether it's surgical or non-surgical, putting them on a hugely restricted eating plan, monitoring their food journals and exercise logs, and keeping the data for a year, after which they can proclaim their program to be a great and wonderful success. Never mind that the year after the patient leaves the weight loss program and has no external accountability or support team, their weight usually returns - "and brings friends."

I cannot help but wonder what the long-term outcome for either surgical, or non-surgical weight loss programs would be if they had a very long-term, graduated program for patients. Maybe six months of intensive education (medical, social and psychological, to include addiction education), followed by another six months of weekly or bi-weekly program attendance during which groups members discuss their successes and challenges, learn healthy coping skills, address addiction difficulties, emotional barriers to success, learn the value of healthy self-talk, receive education about internal motivation and goal-setting, and identify ways to set healthy boundaries with those who might attempt to sabotage their progress. The second year - and for as long as people wanted - they could attend weekly aftercare groups to learn and identify areas in which they need help. I'm guessing the outcomes would be better. And yes – I am going to implement a program such as this! Stay tuned!

In the meantime, let me focus specifically on the topic that professionals at the Centers of Excellence rarely talk about in regard to patient pre-surgical preparation activities. Keep in mind that patients talk about this all the time. It is a topic that is widely discussed and debated at national and international surgical and non-surgical professional medical conferences. It is, perhaps, the greatest reason that people are unable to maintain the behavior modification changes they make while under the careful eye of the medical team. It may be the ultimate reason that a great many people eventually "go back to their old habits." Perhaps it is the primary reason behind the self-sabotaging behaviors in which patients regularly engage. It is most intricately interwoven with the stinkin' thinkin' in the minds and out of the mouths of those suffering from obesity.

This possible barrier to long-term weight management encompasses, and is intertwined with, so many of the emotional and psychological issues that are IGNORED in practice by the medical community. These psychological issues include low self-esteem, negative body image, low self-efficacy, learned helplessness, "victim" mentality, inability to set boundaries, emotional trauma, abuse, neglect, unhealthy family systems, and the list goes on. The single, most devastating, core emotional issue that plagues nearly every person struggling with obesity, an issue not even recognized by most medical professionals, is the SHAME that permeates every cell of our patients beings.

And for many of our patients (again, I did not say all), that shame is shrouded in another disease that patients will readily identify (at least after having weight loss surgery), but the Centers of Excellence and the vast majority of surgeons and medical professionals choose to ignore: FOOD ADDICTION.

While I believe that nearly all patients who struggle with obesity experience shame (the very painful emotion one feels when they believe there is something inherently wrong with who they are), not all persons struggle with food addiction. This book is about those who do have a food addiction, whether a physiological addiction (meaning their brains literally respond to certain substances in a manner similar to other drugs of abuse) or a psychological addiction (meaning people genuinely believe they "need" food to "soothe" or "escape" or "distract" them from life circumstances and/or their feelings).

When all bariatric professionals band together to address food addiction from an in-depth perspective with our bariatric patients, we will likely see much better outcomes. For patients, better outcomes translate to increasing your love and care toward yourself and toward others, and living life fully – on life's terms, at a healthy weight for your body! In other words, living in Recovery from food addiction.

Talk about a fight! You know your struggle with weight has been fraught with one battle after another. You thought life was gonna be all better after weight loss surgery. Now you know there's so much more, including some skirmishes you had no idea you would face after your procedure... Well, damn!

CHAPTER THREE

WHAT COULD THE MATTER BE?

Regain. A very "bad" word in the minds, and on the bodies, of a lot of people. Regain is a scary word, a word that conjures up feelings ranging from unpleasant to nauseating. A word that represents "failure," "self-loathing," "despair," and "hopelessness," particularly if regain occurs following bariatric surgery, which many see as the "last chance," the "hope of hopes." And yet, tragically, there is regain galore following bariatric surgery.

Fortunately, there are scores of people who are able to maintain a healthy weight for the rest of their lives following weight loss surgery. I am a proponent of weight loss surgery as I shared in the previous chapter. Not only can bariatric surgery literally be a physical lifesaver, it also provides opportunities for healing in other ways. As one's physical health improves, people report having more energy to deal with other issues. Oftentimes they start to feel better about themselves, and work to heal their emotional relationship with themselves. Self-esteem increases, self-efficacy surges, and body image improves. These positive changes lead to exercising regularly and eating more nutritious foods, thereby developing a healthy relationship with food. As a person's physical and emotional relationship with himself or herself improves, it often follows that their relationships with others also improve.

Tragically, for those who do experience regain following bariatric surgery, they may give up all hope of winning the immortal "battle of the bulge."

"How many people *do* regain weight after having bariatric surgery?" I honestly believe the accurate answer is, "Who the hell knows for sure?!" If you get your information from the bariatric surgery websites or the governing bodies of bariatric professionals, their "scientific research" will paint quite an optimistic picture. (Remember, they are a business and like all businesses, if they don't have new customers, they will no longer have a business.) Therefore, their information provides amazing outcome statistics. If you read scientific research articles, you will notice that these amazing outcome statistics are the results of studies with patients who are, perhaps, two years out from having had surgery. To which I say, "Well, hip hip hooray! That tells me nothing." For example, I looked up a "scholarly, peer-reviewed article," (meaning it got the thumbs up from medical peers) on long-term outcomes of weight loss surgery. The authors of this article, entitled *Long-Term Outcomes After Bariatric Surgery*, published in 2012, confirmed what I have read in various reports over of the years. These authors stated, "Most of the bariatric surgical literature contains data on short-term follow-up only (< 3 years)." (Citation: O'brien, P. E., MacDonald, L., Anderson, M., Brennan, L., & Brown, W. A. (2013). Long-term outcomes after bariatric surgery: fifteen-year follow-up of adjustable gastric banding and a systematic review of the bariatric surgical literature. *Annals of surgery*, 257(1), 87-94.)

The surgeons with whom I work on a daily basis routinely tell patients that the surgery does its work in the first two years and that most patients will lose the majority of their weight within 12 to 18 months following surgery. Patients are encouraged to use that time to implement the healthy eating and exercise behaviors they will need to maintain for the rest of their lives in order to remain at a healthy weight.

Well, now, if we're sampling people at 24 months following surgery to see how they're doing in terms of weight loss success, I would imagine the results are going to be favorable. Patients are most often enamored with the results they are seeing in terms of weight loss during this "honeymoon stage," and often report not being hungry during this time of physical healing. They tend to be more compliant in the immediate aftermath of surgery because they are motivated by the rapid weight loss and because they haven't felt hungry. I want to shout, "REALLY?!?!? You're reporting weight loss statistics after two years that make it sound to patients like everyone who has bariatric surgery keeps their weight off for a lifetime?! You aren't telling them the entire reality, the facts! You are giving very limited information!!!!! THIS IS PROPAGANDA, hype, advertising, publicity!" It is intentional and it is printed to attract business. For sure, at two years following surgery, the vast majority of patients have maintained all, or most, of their initial weight loss. Great statistics for business, without a doubt!

And I don't blame practices for doing this. Remember, this is a business. This is their business and they want it to thrive.

As a consumer, however, you need to know more of the full story. That story includes regain, much of which may be due to food addiction. Patients need to be made aware of all the factors that can lead to regain during their pre-surgical process. It is the responsibility of those of us involved in this process to impart this information and, at the minimum, provide resources for people to get help. Optimally, bariatric programs would provide ongoing nutritional and psychological services within their practice. And some do! Many thanks to those of you who do!

While searching, I also found an article entitled *Long-Term Impact of Bariatric Surgery on Body Weight, Comorbidities, and Nutritional Status*. These authors reviewed a number of bariatric programs results and concluded: ***"Gastric bypass surgeries lead to substantial weight loss in individuals with morbid obesity. However, significant weight regain occurs over the long term."*** Both findings are true. There is significant weight loss in the early years following bariatric surgery. It is also true that there is often significant weight regain over time for many people. (Citation: Meena Shah, Vinaya Simha, Abhimanyu Garg; Long-Term Impact of Bariatric Surgery on Body Weight, Comorbidities, and Nutritional Status. J Clin Endocrinol Metab 2006; 91 (11): 4223-4231. doi: 10.1210/jc.2006-0557.)

It's difficult to accumulate long-term data for outcomes on weight maintenance and health status following surgery for a number of reasons. Many patients don't follow up with their surgery centers after the first few visits, making data collection impossible. Another problem, which can lead to skewed results, is that those patients for whom there is follow-up data, may only be the ones who are doing well. They may be doing well because they have kept up with their surgeon for annual check-ups, and they may report for annual check-ups because they are doing well. Either way, the information that is available for long-term data collection may only include those patients who continue to do well. This may be a small percentage of the total number of patients who have had bariatric surgery. The research results can be portrayed in such a way as to make it sound like this percentage of patients fairly represents all those who have had bariatric surgery.

In my experience, those patients who reach out seeking "Back on Track" programs have often lapsed in their follow-up appointments, noting they were "embarrassed" or "ashamed" to return to the bariatric center because they had regained weight. Patients I see for evaluations related to a second, "revisional" bariatric procedure report the same information. They didn't come back sooner because they didn't want the doctor to see them "this way."

It is my contention that long-term outcomes following bariatric surgery could improve, perhaps significantly, were we addressing both psychological addiction to food and physiological addiction to food.

PRE-SURGICAL EDUCATION AND COUNSELING, ALONG WITH LONG-TERM ASSISTANCE FOR PATIENTS FOLLOWING BARIATRIC SURGERY FOCUSING ON THE MEDICAL COMMUNITY'S BELOVED "BEHAVIOR MODIFICATION" AS WELL AS THE ESSENTIAL TREATMENT OF THE PSYCHOLOGICAL ISSUES ASSOCIATED WITH OBESITY AND WEIGHT LOSS, TO INCLUDE FOOD ADDICTION, MIGHT VERY WELL IMPROVE LONG-TERM OUTCOMES FOLLOWING BARIATRIC SURGERY.

During the pre-surgical evaluations, I ask each and every patient if they know others who have had weight loss surgery. Nearly everyone does. Some have numerous immediate and extended family members who have had surgery, so more and more "kin," as they say here in the South, are following suit. I've watched over the years as the numbers of employees from the same work institution trickle in, stating that a co-worker who had surgery encouraged them to do the same. This is also true of the many surrounding rural towns in the area I live. We'll have periods of time when one person after another person from a nearby small town will come through our doors.

My follow-up question to the prospective surgical patient is, "How is the person you know who had surgery doing and how long ago did they have their surgery?"

"Oh, they're doing great! She's lost 60 pounds and it's only been 7 months!"

"They look amazing! I think his surgery was last year."

"I barely recognized him! Last time I saw him was last summer at the family reunion. This year he looked like an entirely different person."

"I just can't believe how great she looks! It will be two years ago next month. I know because she was in the hospital on my birthday that year."

"After seeing how great she's done, I knew I had to have surgery. She'll be a year ahead of me, but I know I'll catch up with her weight loss."

Do you hear the common denominator? So, I then follow up with, "Do you know anyone who had the surgery longer ago than the past two or three years?" That's when I get more mixed result responses.

"My aunt had surgery six years ago. She's gained back every pound of the weight she lost. I just can't imagine going through all of this to gain your weight back."

"My husband had surgery five years ago. He lost 150 pounds and I think he's put back on at least 50 pounds. He plans to lose that after I have my surgery. He's even going to do the two-week liquid diet with me before I have my surgery." "How did he regain the weight?" I ask, suspecting she may have some insight, being she's married to the guy.

"Well, you know," she replied rather sheepishly. "After a few years, he started going back to his old ways. At first, he wouldn't touch a potato or eat any bread or pasta. He's going to quit starches again after I have surgery. We're going to follow the guidelines the nutritionist gives us. He said he's learned from his mistakes." "Yep. That's exactly why the nutritionist provides specific guidelines," I say, not sarcastically, but firmly. "Many people think the surgery will take care of their 'weight problem' forever, but for most people, the reality is, you can't have it both ways. You can't eat what you want whenever you want to and maintain a healthy weight. Have you ever discussed the topic of food addiction?"

It's not uncommon for me to hear patient comments such as, "Several people from the plant where I work have had surgery. Some are doing great and it's been years. Some have gained back all of their weight. I'm always surprised by what I see those fellas eating. I didn't think you were supposed to eat certain things after surgery." I affirm what he's just said. "You're right. When you go through the nutritionist's class before surgery, and when you meet with her after surgery, you'll learn that a healthy way of eating for a post bariatric patient is different than for people who go on specific types of 'diets.' We encourage people to eat small portions of healthy foods, avoiding added sugars and avoiding unnecessary, unhealthy carbohydrates while taking in healthy sources of protein."

I hear a lot about weight regain, whether it is told to me by patients describing their weight histories during pre-surgical evaluations, by people at a social gathering chatting about weight problems, or when I do evaluations for people desiring a "revision" surgery, a second weight loss surgery because they regained all, or a good portion, of the weight they lost following their initial bariatric procedure. By far the most frequent reason for weight regain is "I went back to my old habits." Not to presume to know what specifically those habits were, although I could, by this point in time, make a darn good guess, I always ask, "What specific habits were those for you?" You don't need to be a psychologist or have conducted over 4000 pre-surgical evaluations (yes, I have), to know what responses go on the top responses list. Although, if I were on Family Feud again, I wouldn't be able to come up with even one, as evidenced by my pathetic (but truly fun and hysterical) performance when I was up there on stage with Mr. Harvey! Regarding the question of unhealthy "old habits" that lead to weight regain, I most often hear:

- I started eating a lot of carbs again.
- I got tired of eating the same things.
- I stopped exercising.
- I resumed drinking sweet tea (soda, fancy coffee drinks).
- I stopped planning meals.
- I quit measuring portions.
- I started going out to eat a lot/went back to driving through fast food chains.
- I quit drinking water.
- I reintroduced sugar into my diet.
- I bought a lot of processed food at the grocery store.
- Etc. etc. etc.

You know what I am much more interested in than what the old habits are? The reason people return to them. THAT gives me insight to what's going on for this person and what they might need to help them. "What happens/happened that you returned to your "old habits?" (I refer to these responses, by the way, as "surface responses." You'll learn why in just a minute). Common surface responses include:

- I got too busy.
- I care for everyone but me.
- I don't know.
- Food calls to me.
- I just don't have time.
- I lost motivation.
- My mother (or father, or sister) got sick (died).
- Work got too busy.
- I started going to the grocery store instead of having someone else go.
- I had no competition, which always inspires me to lose weight.
- If I start with sugar, I don't seem able to quit.
- I have to run kids all over and we only have time for fast food.
- I felt deprived.
- I couldn't think about anything but food all day long.
- I started smoking again when I was dieting and I don't want to smoke.
- I missed ice cream.
- It's too hard working swing shift to stay on a good eating schedule.
- The rest of my family was eating different foods and I hated cooking two meals.

For those persons who have had a bariatric surgery, have regained weight and are seeking a revision surgery (a second weight loss surgery), in addition to many of the responses listed above, their reasons for returning to "old habits" may include:

- I didn't like the attention I got from people when I lost weight.
- I didn't know who I was when I lost so much weight.

Literally, not one time in the 14 years I've worked in this field, have I had anyone tell me, "I returned to my old habits because I'm addicted to food." And yet, so many post-ops readily identify themselves as food addicts when asked. WHEN ASKED! Hmmm... there may be something to that! (If you are a medical professional, take note.)

In chapter two I stated that obesity "isn't about the food." Let me give a preview (foreshadowing I think they call it in novels) of my reason for saying that obesity isn't about the food. It's related to all of this regain, which I think we can all agree is a routine occurrence for those who have fought weight problems for years. It seems to me that if "solving" obesity were about eating the right foods in correct portion sizes and exercising on a regular basis via "behavior modification," which is what most medical and surgical programs are based upon, then once a person loses the weight and knows these "answers," there would be no regain were it not for psychological and/or biological reasons. Hence, my re-stating that obesity isn't just about the food. It's only partly about the food. And honestly, I think everyone pretty much knows this, although the medical community apparently either doesn't want to acknowledge it, or simply doesn't want to deal with it.

The patients know, however. Every day I see comments on social media that underscore patients' understanding of the need for psychological attention following weight loss surgery. Here are a few postings patients posted just today:

- The brain work is so difficult and at times feels impossible.
- Head battles are constant and never really go away.

Before I get deep into these psychological issues, including Food Addiction, let's review the main factors associated with obesity, which were listed in Chapter Two.

The list of factors contributing to obesity includes the following (remember, I added Addiction to this list; the rest come from nationally renowned medical sites):

- Genetics
- Culture and Environment
- Metabolism
- Illness and Medications
- Sleep

- Personal Behaviors
- Psychological Aspects
- *Addiction*

I say it's pointless to spend a lot of time, attention or money on the things in this list you can't really influence in your present life. On the other hand, it makes a great deal of sense to put effort into areas where you can influence your weight, your health and your ability to live life fully.

There's little you can do as an adult to alter your genetic history regarding family predisposition for obesity. What's the point in focusing on that as you work to lose weight and keep it off? The best thing to do in terms of your genetics is accept them. That does not, mind you, mean liking the fact that "every woman on my mother's side of the family for the past four generations has been obese." It means accepting that you, if you are a female in that family, are likely predisposed to that same genetic pattern. You can be ticked off all day long about it if you want to. But that's not going to help much, unless you are the type of person who gets motivated by anger. As is true in so much of life... it is what it is. Accept that you have fat genes. It means you'll probably have to work harder to maintain a healthy weight than another person might. That's what I mean when I talk about "life on life's terms." There's not much you can do to change that. So let's put our focus and effort elsewhere.

How about culture and environment? "I grew up in an Italian family where food is love! The men and women in my family know how to cook and to cook well! We celebrate everything with food. And there's something to celebrate in our family, it appears, every day!" "I'm from a traditional Hispanic household. We eat rice with beans, scooped up in a tortilla every day." "I'm Asian. Rice is a staple in my world."

OK! That's what you were raised with. You likely had very little choice about what you were fed as a child. You do have a choice today. Personal behaviors as an adult require making healthy food choices and healthy portions IF you want to maintain a healthy weight for YOUR body given YOUR genetic reality. You can change generations of tradition if you choose to. It depends on what you want and how much effort you are willing to put into it.

And so it goes. Metabolism is clearly different for each person. There are ways to boost your metabolism, such as drinking ice water, which you can implement in your life. You also need to accept the fact (deal with life on life's terms) that your metabolism may be slower than other people's. Once you accept facts, then you can make choices based on reality. In this case, if you have a slow metabolism, you won't be able to eat as much as persons with a higher metabolism. It sucks – and you can have a temper tantrum about it (which might actually be good for your mental health), but temper tantrums and refusal to make adjustments to your food intake certainly won't help you get weight off or maintain a healthy weight!

As for illnesses and medications, there may be times when you opt to take a medication known to cause weight gain because your health depends on it. Your personal choices are again an important factor in such cases. You may have to reduce caloric intake and/or increase exercise while you are on medications that are known to increase weight. Them's the facts. Deal with them head on and make healthy personal choices accordingly.

For most people, sleep – when and how much – is also a personal behavior choice. Not so for others who suffer with sleep disorders or swing shifts. Do what you can with your medical professional to get the best sleep possible and make it a healthy personal behavior to get close to 8 hours of sleep at a time. Sleep – it's proven to be related to maintaining a healthy weight. So again, it's up to you!

And now… here it is. Two critical aspects of obesity, two areas that you can greatly influence. Both are largely culpable in relation to weight issues, particularly regain. ***Psychological Aspects*** related to weight loss. And ***Food Addiction***. The sadly overlooked, ignored, mistreated outlaws to medical science. You and I, however, know the importance of providing what is needed for more long-term weight loss success: psychological care and addiction treatment via pre- and post-op therapy classes, therapeutic groups and individual care.

Now, now, bariatric physicians and program coordinators, before you get your undies in a wad, I know that you are providing what "they say" is essential for a bariatric Center of Excellence. So what. It's not the patients who are determining what those criteria are. It's a group of medical business people. And what they require is not enough.

A major THANK YOU to those practices who go above and beyond what the COE requirements are. THANK YOU to those who have mental health practitioners in your practices, who offer therapeutic groups in addition to the mandated Support Groups (which are great but don't often cover psychological issues). THANK YOU for using video series designed to better prepare patients for what to expect after surgery in the psychological and social arenas. THANK YOU for doing your very best to "DO NO HARM" to your patients. I have the pleasure of working with, and knowing many of you. I'm truly impressed by your dedication to your patients and their mental and physical wellbeing.

REGAIN: WHAT THE MATTERS ARE

What could the matter be? Why is it that so many people regain weight in this battle with obesity? There are clearly some medical issues related to weight regain. Those medical issues are complex and I am not qualified to explain them. I can, however, refer you to a wonderful author who does that extremely well, Vera Tarman, M.D. In her truly amazing book about food addiction titled Food Junkies (by Vera Tarman and Philip Werdell), Dr. Tarman explains the science behind obesity and weight regain. She also explains the science of food addiction. Thank you, Dr. Tarman for doing this, as I don't want to go anywhere near attempting that.

I am qualified, on the other hand, to discuss the psychological/emotional issues related to obesity. And I am qualified to discuss food addiction. Although there are some people who have a food addiction and may not have a lot of the psychological/emotional issues that often accompany both obesity and addiction, in my experience, those who have any addiction have at least some complementary psychological/emotional issues. Therefore, for ease of discussion, I am going to discuss them simultaneously. Hang in there with me. I promise to clarify further as we move along.

Let's return again to the "surface responses" patients provide when asked, "What happened that you returned to unhealthy 'old habits' and experienced weight regain?" I have listed examples of their responses below. Beneath their surface responses, I provide some possible psychological interpretations, which suggest what the real (psychological/emotional) needs of the patient may be. This list is partial and there are likely many additional possibilities.

Here we go. Patients say, in response to the question, "What happened that you returned to unhealthy 'old habits' and regained weight?" in these ways:

"I GOT TOO BUSY," OR "I DON'T HAVE TIME TO EAT RIGHT AND TO EXERCISE," OR "WORK GOT CRAZY."

Possible interpretations:

- "I don't count."
- "I'm not as important as others."
- "I don't care enough about me."
- "If I stay overly busy, I won't have to address my own needs, care for myself, or pay attention to my needs or wants. I don't want to look inside myself."
- "I have ADD/ADHD."
- "I may have a food addiction."

"I TAKE CARE OF EVERYONE BUT MYSELF."

Possible interpretations:

- "I was told directly or indirectly by words and actions from parents/siblings/teachers/coaches/kids and/or others that I didn't matter and I believe it."
- "I don't count."
- "I'm not as important as others."
- "I don't care enough about me."
- "I may have a food addiction."

"I DON'T KNOW WHY I RETURN TO OLD HABITS."

Possible interpretations:

- "I am not at all aware of psychological issues and truly don't have any conscious reason for why I do what I do or don't do."
- "I don't want to think about the possible reasons."
- "I want to avoid myself, my thoughts, my feelings and my behavior because I don't like what I'll see."
- "I may have a food addiction."

FOOD CALLS TO ME.

Possible interpretations:

- "I have a need for distraction for things currently going on in

my life and food provides that."
- "I'm not happy with me/others/past issues/feelings and food tells me it can make me feel better."
- "I hear things other people do not."
- "I may have a food addiction."

"I LOST MOTIVATION," OR "I HAD NO COMPETITION."

Possible interpretations:
- "I'm not doing this for me."
- "I like competition but I'm not that interested in myself."
- "I don't matter."
- "I may have a food addiction."

"I STARTED GOING TO THE GROCERY STORE INSTEAD OF HAVING SOMEONE ELSE GO."

Possible interpretations:
- "I missed my friend, food, and going to the store gave me an excuse to get what I want."
- "Food serves me in some way (makes me feel better, helps me avoid feelings, help me fight loneliness, etc.) and I don't want to deal with those things. I'd rather struggle with food. It's easier."
- "I may have a food addiction."

"IF I START WITH SUGAR, I DON'T SEEM ABLE TO QUIT."

Possible interpretations:
- "I have no off switch."
- "I may have a food addiction."

"I HAVE TO RUN KIDS ALL OVER AND WE ONLY HAVE TIME FOR FAST FOOD."

Possible interpretations:
- "My weight/my self is not a priority."
- See possible interpretations above for: "I got too busy," or "I don't have time to eat right and to exercise," or "Work got crazy."
- "I may have a food addiction."

I FELT DEPRIVED WHEN I WAS ON A DIET.

Possible interpretations:

- "I have needs that are not being met."
- "I feel empty inside."
- "I was very restricted in the past."
- "I need ... freedom? Space? Personal choices?"
- "I had very little in my past."
- "I may have a food addiction."

"I STARTED SMOKING AGAIN WHEN I WAS DIETING AND I DON'T WANT TO SMOKE."

Possible interpretations:

- "I need something to avoid dealing with…
  - reality?
  - feelings?
  - unresolved issues?
- "I may be an addict playing whack-a-mole addiction."

I MISSED ICE CREAM.

Possible interpretations:

- "I need something to avoid dealing with…
  - reality?
  - feelings?
  - unresolved issues?
- "I have a need for distraction for things currently going on in my life and food provides that."
- "I'm not happy with me/others/past issues/feelings and food tells me it can make me feel better."
- "I may have a food addiction."

IT'S TOO HARD WORKING SWING SHIFT TO STAY ON A GOOD EATING SCHEDULE.

Possible interpretations:

- "I'm not worth the effort to put into doing what I need to do for my health."
- "I don't count."
- "I may have a food addiction."

punishment, or a psychological escape. Food addiction treatment includes additional steps (the topic of the remaining chapters), but here's a summary of the healing process:

- Go beneath the surface answer to "What happened that you regained weight in the past after losing weight?"

- That response will reveal the person's "underlying," or genuine emotional/psychological needs. In other words, "I regained my weight because .... _____. " The because (whatever it is) tells us the problem(s). For example:

  - "I regained my weight because I'm so busy with the kids and work and simply don't have time," **(the surface response)** which translates to, "I regained my weight because I don't think I matter to others and I don't really matter that much to myself" **(genuine issue)**. *The person needs* to heal the relationship they have with themselves. By learning they are important, they can begin to treat themselves with the same amount of love and care with which they treat others. With help, this can transfer to caring for one's own health via food and exercise. Unless they learn to know they matter and are as important as others, they'll not likely treat themselves any better than in the past. (Did you address this at your bariatric center?)

  - "I regained my weight because I take care of so many others," **(the surface response)** which translates to, "I continue to hear negative things about myself that others said to me throughout my life. Food distracts me from remembering and feeling" **(genuine issue)**. *The person needs* to deal with their feelings related to negative comments made to them in the past. More importantly, *the person needs* to become aware of, and then REFUSE to talk to/treat him/herself with harsh words or behavior. This is difficult to do and takes the rest of their lives to improve upon. It also requires the help and support of others who point out harsh self-talk and unhealthy behaviors. As their words and actions toward self improve, they are more likely to treat themselves more kindly in terms of how they eat, exercise, and care for their bodies.

- "I regained my weight because I felt deprived on diets," **(the surface response)** which translates to, "I don't want to remember/feel/think about how poor we were as children and how my father drank instead of buying food for us" (replace with any past problems, past thoughts, past feelings, losses = **genuine issue**). *The person needs* to address and grieve the feelings and losses from the past. They then need to focus on the fact they are no longer victims of other people's behavior or circumstances. They must make the decision to become dependable to themselves. Again, this is long-term work and requires the support and assistance of others, but can make a huge impact on a person's life, how they treat themselves, how they eat and otherwise care for their bodies, and can also help improve other relationships in their lives.

- "I regained my weight because I didn't like how people looked at me when I lost weight," **(the surface issue)** which translates to "I was molested by a neighbor and never told anyone. In my family, we were never taught how to identify feelings, talk about feelings in healthy ways, set healthy boundaries, or communicate effectively. In recent years, food was a way to avoid remembering, feeling or having to deal with others" **(genuine issue)**. *The person needs* to work with a trained professional to express their thoughts and feelings about their abuse in order to heal from it. *The person also needs* to learn to identify how they feel, how to express those feelings in appropriate ways, and how to set healthy boundaries for themselves. They will likely need to grieve and learn they are no longer a victim. They can make healthy choices for themselves in all areas of life, to include food selection, portion size, and what type of exercise to do. These are terribly difficult things to learn and utilize on a regular basis, but they are very do-able. These things take time, effort and commitment.

Hopefully in healing the psychological issues, the patient will heal their relationship with self. As this healing takes place, the patient will no longer treat their body or themselves poorly through unhealthy food behaviors and a lack of (or abuse of) exercise. In addition, they will be better able to follow through with those necessary (but insufficient) behavior modification tools. Bottom line?

The healing can be done. The healing of inner issues can and does transfer to treating oneself in a kinder, more loving way. This includes caring more for one's physical health, which results in being better able to sustain a healthy weight.

Remember how I referred earlier to the behavior modification aspects of weight loss (choosing healthy foods, eating the right serving size, exercising) as being necessary but insufficient for sustained weight loss? Now you know why. There are so many underlying psychological/emotional issues that interfere with one's willingness/ability to follow through with those behaviors.

If you are familiar with my work, I refer to the behavior modification aspects as the Gotta Do Ems (see References). These are the behaviors you gotta do if you're going to keep weight off. The other thing people need to do is address whatever underlying issues get in the way of following through with the Gotta Do Ems. Again, these underlying issues can include not believing you matter, having unresolved feelings related to prior loss, abuse, or neglect, not knowing how to set healthy boundaries, not knowing how to communicate assertively (as opposed to aggressively or passive-aggressively), and/or having an addiction to food/eating.

THEN WHY DOESN'T EVERYONE HEAL

Naturally, there isn't just one answer. Here are several reasons people don't heal their underlying issues (the real problems):

- They don't know they have them (think they are "fine" just the way they are).

- They protect themselves from acknowledging how much damage their underlying issues have caused them (and others) through "defense mechanisms" such as denial, minimization, screaming, blaming, arguing to keep themselves from seeing their flaws.

- Working through the emotional/psychological work is difficult, painful, frightening at times, and can take a very long period of time.

From my perspective, it is our responsibility as adults to get help for whatever the matter is. If it is our physical health that needs tending to, then tend to it. If it is emotional health that needs assistance, get on it. If you have a food addiction, continue reading as the rest of the book is devoted to how to deal with that.

WHEN FOOD ADDICTION IS PRESENT

If you suspect you have an addiction to food, then nearly all of the above genuine issues (not believing you matter, not caring enough about yourself, having experienced some degree of unresolved grief/loss, having experienced some degree of neglect or abuse, not having learned to identify and deal with feelings in the most appropriate ways, not having learned to set healthy boundaries, not having learned healthy communication skills, and ultimately neglecting and abusing yourself in the present) applies to you.

How do I know? Personal experience with addiction, 10 years of college, and 25 years of professional experience in the field. Trust me.

Before you scoff and close the book for good, ask yourself how you are feeling at this very minute. If you have ever referred to yourself as a food addict, does this last section scare you? Anger you? Disgust you? Intrigue you? Most people don't like thinking of themselves as a person who: does not believe they matter, doesn't care enough about themself, has unresolved grief/loss, has experienced neglect or abuse, hasn't learned to identify and deal with feelings in appropriate ways, has not learned to set healthy boundaries, does not have healthy communication skills, and as someone who neglects and abuses themself.

Read on and you'll understand.

By the way, does weight loss surgery, a procedure done to your guts, treat any of those issues? Hmmm… what *could* the matter be?

CHAPTER FOUR

THE "A" WORD

Who wants to be an addict? Did your hand shoot up in the air as you finished reading those words? Who wants to be a millionaire? I'm guessing more people would opt for millionaire than addict! Addict. It just sounds ugly. Dirty. Like someone who is pathetic and hopeless. La-hoooooo-ser! The big L.

Well, I'm a recovering addict and those negative words certainly don't describe me! In fact, I am happy to say that I am now a "Grateful Recovering Addict." This is a phrase I would hear at AA meetings nearly 30 years ago when I first started attending. I could not fathom what those people were saying! What was there to be grateful for, being an addict, recovering or otherwise? If you stick around long enough, do some intense work on healing yourself from the inside out, then you'll know from experience what it means to be a Grateful Recovering Addict. That is, if you're actually an addict...

I'll give you a visual that might help you understand what I mean when I say "addict." When your world is consumed with, or controlled by food, weight, alcohol, spending, sex, gambling, or anything that causes problems in your life, that you wish you could stop but haven't been able to, you're living in addiction. It's like living in a world that is covered by an ugly, itchy, tattered brown blanket. Everything in your world seems brown. Colorless. You go through life and you have everything you need to be functional, but life is dull, covered by a layer of beige gunk. Even if your world is full of chaos, it's drab. You're existing. The heavy, burdensome coating of yuck is always there. It covers everything and there is no escape.

Picture this. You're existing in a drab, perhaps chaotic world in which you are obsessed with food: eating food, thinking about food, watching the food network, scouring recipes, posting pictures of your food on social media, drooling over other people's pictures of food on social media, snacking, eyeing other people's food, reading restaurant menus, and maybe even dreaming about food. Food rules your world.

One day you are drawn to a very large lake. You can see across the lake, but it is a very far distance. The distance is not so great, however, that you cannot see that things are different over on the other side of the lake. You see... what is that over there? Whatever it is, it's not brown! Why, you see green! Yes! The trees over there are green? And what is that in the sky? It's another color! Blue! And there are white, fluffy clouds over there! You look up toward the heavens on your side of the lake and what you see is a brown sky with brown clouds. Depressing.

You peer across the water, searching for a glimpse of other colorful sights. Lo and behold, you marvel at what you see! Although the objects are too far away to see clearly, you definitely see pink things! And yellow things! Why, it seems like everything on that side of the lake is vibrant! Colorful. Alive. Exciting. You want to go THERE!

Home you go as fast as you can to your computer and search, "lake at the edge of town with colorful life on the other side." And up pops a picture of the lake, from the exact vantage point you experienced it! The side you live on is brown, drab and dreary. The other side is bright, glorious, and energetic. You notice, as you scan the various pictures of the lake, that the color of the lake water itself changes from one shore to the other. On the side where you exist, the water is murky, muddy, and ominous. The hues change across the distance of the lake. The closer to the other shore, the water becomes green and blue, sparkling, clear and inviting. You NEED to go THERE! To live on the other side of this lake.

You search for the name of the lake on the screen in front of you. Ah – there it is: Lake Hælan. That's an odd name. You search for more. Here's what you discover:

> "Lake Hælan is a body of water with curative properties. Passage on foot through Lake Hælan restores a person to their original state of wholeness. A walk through the water revitalizes people, and transforms them to their original state of soundness and wellness. The healing riches embedded in the lake water awaken that which has been damaged in one's mind, body and spirit. However, the healing journey through the lake can be treacherous, is painful, and is, overall very frightening. For these reasons, few venture to make the journey, opting instead for the safety and security of a life that is familiar, although far from desirable. Although wanting to live more fully on the healthy side of the lake, many people continue to exist in a constant state of boredom, misery, anger, resentment, victimization or feigned happiness on the drab, unhealthy side of the lake. Those who courageously opt to make the journey open themselves to experiencing feelings related to unresolved past grief, fear, loss, neglect, abuse, ridicule, and bullying from others. They painfully but clearly see the damage they continue to cause themselves (and others) through harsh self-talk, self-abuse, self-neglect. They see how addiction to food, substances, other people, shopping or other substances/behaviors has caused problems for their health, their sense of self, and in their relationships with others. Many a curious soul tiptoes into the lake only to run back to the safety of the familiarity of their life mired in addiction. The bravest of the brave move forward, making their way to the center of the lake where they find themselves completely covered in the shame that is the shroud of addiction. If a person turns back toward the brown shore, they remain stuck. They are mired in the awareness that they are their own worst enemy. They have the option to make changes but they are too afraid to do so. They remain bogged down in a life of inner shame, feeling they are less worthy than others, feeling unable to make the changes they wish they could."

Wow! After reading this on your computer screen, you pause and think about your relationship with food. You recognize the cloak that is the obsession with food. You relate to how your obsession with food prevents you from living more fully. You know you have made attempts in the past to free yourself from the chains binding you to food but you have not been freed. You recognize the discomfort associated with trying to live without food as the center of your world. You have opted, every time you have tried to get free from the bondage of food, to return to a life ruled by food. It is easier to live there than to go through the pain of change. The world of food is a familiar (and safe) place to you. Regardless of how unhappy a place it might be.

Interesting! Since you were able to find this information on Lake Hælan with the simple click of a mouse, being obsessed with food is clearly not unique to you. You *do* have a choice about remaining there or leaving! You **can** heal. Hmmm… what to do?

Do you stay and live your familiar brown life where food is miserably all consuming? Or do you move forward to an unfamiliar place, knowing that the journey may be painful but the reward great?

Those who are committed to living on the colorful side of the lake trust that life there is worth the journey. They accept the past and the whoever and the whatever that caused them pain during their life. They accept they were born with a brain susceptible to addiction. They accept the pain they have experienced and the pain they continue to cause themselves (and others) by not moving toward the hope and the help that exists. They move toward the beauty of the opposite shore, knowing they can leave the pain and shame of addiction at the bottom of the lake.

With every inch forward toward the brightness, hope is palpable. Adventurers feel a literal transformation within their body, their mind, and their spirit. They KNOW with certainty that they if they continue on, they can leave the drab side of the lake for good. They no longer need to stay stuck in the misery. They courageously face the unpleasant feelings that live inside them. They wade through the murkiness of the water and the muddiness of their addiction-rooted thoughts, the unhealthy thinking that held rational thought hostage and prevented positive thoughts from taking root. They let go of the substances and behaviors that held them captive on the dismal, dreary side of life. They face their fears and determinedly make their way through the lake, trusting that life on the other side is worth the perilous, painful journey. Why do they trust this? Because if they look carefully enough, they can see the many people on the shore waving them forward, offering encouragement and support. Surely, those people have successfully navigated their way through Lake Hælan. They are happy. They are joyous. They are free.

On the healthy, colorful side of life awaits the fullness of life and people living as we were meant to live: confidently, securely, able to accept life with its up and downs in healthy ways, able to brush aside negative thoughts, willing to share our unique gifts with others. The people living in color laugh, cry, and love. They live fully. They are continuously healing the relationship they have with themselves. They believe they are as worthy as others of happiness and joy and good health, nurturing food, physical exercise and taking time for self. They know and accept that life has hardships but they learn to deal with them in healthy ways. They learn to communicate in healthy ways and to set healthy boundaries for themselves. They choose, by coming to the colorful side of the lake, to associate with other healthy people, to support one another, to continue to learn, and to accept the good and the difficult parts of life. These people refuse to engage in behaviors or partake of substances that are harmful to them. They know peace. They feel joy.

These are the Grateful Recovering Addicts.

HOW BADLY DO YOU WANT TO LIVE THERE?

You gotta want that life pretty bad to get it. At this point, you might be thinking, "Well, I'm probably not even an addict. My life isn't that bad. I have a lot of good people and things in my life. I'm happy and if I'm not, I often pretend I am. And I sure don't wanna go through a lake filled with crap. I don't even like water."

Perhaps it is time to describe what an addict actually is. I'll let you know at the outset, however, there is no way out of addiction but to go through the healing process. In other words, if you are an addict, or even if you're not, but your struggle with food or people or life has you living in a murky place, the only way to arrive at a place of living fully and at peace is to go through some pain.

WHAT IS AN ADDICT?

Let's just go ahead and get the big, hairy medical definition of addiction out of the way. Then we'll talk about real life stuff that will likely paint a clearer picture.

Here is a scientific definition of addiction as defined by the American Society of Addiction Medicine (ASAM). Just so you know who/what ASAM is: "ASAM, founded in 1954, is a professional society representing over 4,000 physicians, clinicians and associated professionals in the field of addiction medicine. ASAM is dedicated to increasing access and improving the quality of addiction treatment, educating physicians and the public, supporting research and prevention, and promoting the appropriate role of physicians in the care of patients with addiction." (from http://www.asam.org/about-us)

Their "short definition" of addiction is this:

> *"Addiction is a primary, chronic disease of brain reward, motivation, memory and related circuitry. Dysfunction in these circuits leads to characteristic biological, psychological, social and spiritual manifestations. This is reflected in an individual pathologically pursuing reward and/or relief by substance use and other behaviors."*

So what that says is addiction is a disease involving a lot of different brain processes, which affect the addict's thoughts, feelings and behaviors in various areas of their lives (social, emotional, spiritual, and biological). When under the influence of their drug, addicts often lack good judgment, make poor decisions and engage in behaviors that go against their own values. The addict's substance or behavior is used either to make them feel good (the reward, the high, the escape) or to help them avoid feeling bad (as in using drugs to ease a depressed state or to avoid feeling withdrawal symptoms). A chronic disease means the disease is incurable but can be treated.

ASAM goes on to say, *"Addiction is characterized by inability to consistently abstain, impairment in behavioral control, craving, diminished recognition of significant problems with one's behaviors and interpersonal relationships, and a dysfunctional emotional response. Like other chronic diseases, addiction often involves cycles of relapse and remission. Without treatment or engagement in recovery activities, addiction is progressive and can result in disability or premature death."*

This says that without treatment, addicts have trouble staying away from their drug or addictive behavior for long periods of time. Addicts experience uncontrollable cravings for the substance or behavior. They often struggle to recognize the problems related to and caused by their addictions. They are in denial that they have a problem. This of course, often negatively affects their personal relationships. The addiction cycle often includes "falling off the wagon," as well as periods of doing well. The effects of addiction worsen over time and if the addiction is not treated, the person can become disabled or die prematurely.

Believe it or not, ASAM has a much longer definition of addiction that I will not include. However, there are some very interesting things I think you might want to know included in their long definition. I will highlight those for you. (You're welcome!):

Addiction affects numerous brain reward structures which alter motivation, overthrowing or undermining healthy, self-care related behaviors.

- In other words, because addiction involves brain systems, addicts don't always take the best care of their health and they struggle to maintain motivation to follow through with the behaviors necessary to remain abstinent from the substance or behavior.

- Food addicts, in spite of verbalizing a desire to make healthy changes, struggle to follow through with those healthy behaviors. This is, in part, due to brain systems being affected by their addiction to food.

The memory of prior experiences with addictive substances/behaviors triggers cravings or engagement in addictive behaviors.

- Being with people or in places that remind you of when you "used" your substance or behavior can trigger cravings or using.

- It's nearly impossible to completely avoid food triggers. Commercials for food are on the TV, the radio, social media and billboards. Food is omnipresent in our culture. People in Recovery from food addiction need a very strong support network for when they struggle with triggers.

Several brain functions in addiction result in "altered impulse control, altered judgment, and the dysfunctional pursuit of rewards (which is often experienced by the affected person as a desire to 'be normal')."

- Altered brain functioning can result in difficulty delaying gratification and can lead to spontaneous behaviors that may be deleterious.
- Eating before thinking about the consequences, and choosing unhealthy food options in spite of having adequate knowledge may be due to the brain dysfunction related to addiction.

"Genetic factors account for about half of the likelihood that an individual will develop addiction."

- If addiction runs in your family, you are more prone to being an addict.
- A food addict may have family members who are "drug addicts" or "alcoholics," and yet the addiction genes are there. A food addict's drug of choice is food (most often sugar and simple carbohydrates).

"Environmental factors interact with the person's biology." This affects how much influence the genetic factors will have.

- Things in a person's environment (where you live, who you live with, what goes on inside the home, etc.) affect how much impact the genetic factors will have on whether or not one becomes an addict.
- If a person with a genetic predisposition for addiction is raised in a chaotic dysfunctional environment, the addiction genes are more likely to "turn on" than if they are raised in a calm, stable, nurturing environment.

How resilient a person is (based on the type of parenting they received or on life experience) can also affect how much of the genetic predisposition will show up in addictive behavior.

- In other words, just because a person has a genetic predisposition to addiction does not mean they will necessarily behave as an addict. Healthy parenting and/or healthy life experiences can prevent an inherited predisposition for addiction from showing up and playing out.

ASAM also states that addiction involves how a person thinks and feels. The behavior and interactions of addicts with family members, friends, and coworkers is often negatively impacted by their addiction. Addicts come from a deep place of negativity, which can't help from seeping into their thoughts and behaviors at times. So you see, addiction truly does affect all areas of a person's life. And the addict often cannot see how their addiction is harming them or the people in their lives. This can make the disease pretty darned hard to treat!

OTHER DEFINITIONS OF ADDICTION

Various authors and professionals commonly refer to addiction in the following ways: a brain disease, a spiritual disease, a family illness, a social disease, and a bio-psycho-social disease. I believe addiction affects all areas of a person's life, which may hit painfully close to home for you, especially when we talk about food addiction in action in the next chapter.

There are a handful of professionals I especially admire for their work the field of addiction. Some of these professionals are psychiatrists. For those of you who confuse psychiatry and psychology, psychiatrists are medical doctors/physicians, who have been through medical school and can prescribe medications. They attend four years of college, followed by four years of medical school, followed by three or four years of residency (additional training). Psychologists, like myself, are PhD's who engage in "talk therapy" and who generally cannot prescribe medications. We attend four years of college, four to six years of graduate school, and complete a one-year internship.

Gabor Mate is a Canadian psychiatrist (medical doctor) who works with patients suffering from mental illness, drug addiction and HIV, or all three. In his book, <u>In the Realm of Hungry Ghosts: Close Encounters with Addiction</u>, Dr. Mate says that addiction is a brain disease, but for addition to occur, two conditions must be met: 1) a susceptible individual and 2) stress. A person susceptible to addiction, according to Dr. Mate, would be one who likely has a genetic predisposition for addiction, whose childhood was stressful for any number of reasons (poverty, an ill family member, an addicted family member, neglect, abuse, etc.), and who is experiencing stress in the present. "Addiction is all about lack of peace. It's all about internal unrest. It's all about disconnection from the self... a desperate emptiness," says Dr. Mate.

John Bradshaw, who passed away in May of 2016, was a brilliant educator, theologian, and counselor. He was abandoned by an alcoholic father who was himself abandoned by his father. In one of his many books, <u>Bradshaw On: The Family, A New Way of Creating Solid Self-Esteem</u>, Mr. Bradshaw stated, "Our addictions and compulsivities are our mood alterers. They are what we develop when we grow numb. They are our ways of being alive and our ways of managing our feelings... Addictions provide relief."

<u>Adult Children: The Secrets of Dysfunctional Families</u> by John Friel and Linda Friel is one of my all-time favorite books. Reading it helped me understand my life more clearly, and lead to dramatic positive changes for myself and for my family. When I was in my Master's program, I had the honor and privilege to participate as a group co-leader in one of Dr. Friel's weekend workshops. I had, years earlier, participated as a patient in two of his other workshops. The Friels' state, "In the narrowest sense, an addiction is a physiological dependence on some substance, in which the dependence has got out of control and is affecting the daily functioning of the addict in some pretty serious ways."

Tennie McCarty agrees. "It is this loss of control that defines addiction." Tennie wrote an amazing book, titled <u>Shades of Hope: How to Treat Your Addiction to Food</u>. Tennie, herself, is a recovering food addict who runs a food addiction treatment program in Texas. She hosted a program on Oprah's OWN Network called *Addicted to Food*. It was an amazing, true-to-life series showing the power of food addiction and the destruction it had caused to the personal, professional, and interpersonal relationships of the women at the treatment center. I feared it was going to be another sensationalized, over-the-top "reality" show like so many others designed to obtain ratings rather than to spread the truth. Not this one, buddy! It was R.E.A.L! About addiction, Tennie says, "If you can't just take it or leave it, then you are probably addicted to it."

Vera Tarman is a Canadian psychiatrist and co-author of a must-read for food addicts titled, <u>Food Junkies</u>. Dr. Tarman says, "What distinguishes addictive behaviour is its extreme nature: the degree to which a person is compelled to eat, is obsessed with eating. Some people are merely tempted, giving in occasionally. Willpower works for them." Willpower is not enough for food addicts. Dr. Tarman continues, "As humans, we all sit somewhere on a continuum, with desire at one end and addiction at the other. Some of us eat for healthy reasons – for nutrition, as part of social interaction and, yes, for pleasure. Others eat because they are driven by an insatiable need to eat, regardless of hunger or health. A need that is beyond willpower or common sense. It becomes a need that is disconnected from nutrition, interaction, or even pleasure. When an eating behavior leads to a self-destructive end point, when there is a desire to eat that has no 'stop' switch, that trajectory points to the dynamic of addiction."

Keith Ablow is a psychiatrist, author and news personality. He wrote another of my all time favorite reads: <u>Living the Truth: Transform Your Life Through the Power of Insight and Honesty</u>. Do yourself a favor and sit down with that book for a spell! I love that Dr. Ablow, a medical doctor, makes the statement, "At the heart of this and all misguided clinical approaches to addiction is the belief that addicts have broken brains, not deep emotional wounds. I know otherwise." Now, I'm certain there is brain circuitry involved in addiction, as too much research has shown that. And I'm sure Dr. Ablow knows all about that brain stuff, as well. What he is saying, however, is in order to treat addictions, we're not going to do brain surgery. We have to talk about our emotional pain. He's a wise man, that one!

You know why I think most people don't get the help they need for addictions? Because they are afraid. Afraid of feeling. And they are afraid of their feelings because they work so hard (through their addictions) to avoid feeling. That's part of what addictions "do" for us and why we cling to them for so long.

Here's a little more foreshadowing of what's to come in this book… people are afraid to feel their feelings because a lot of why they are "using" food or drugs or shopping is to avoid dealing with issues from the past. We all carry "stuff" with us from the past. Some people were fortunate enough to have adults help them through difficult times and so they have left the past in the past. Others were left alone to try to cope with issues too big for children or adolescents to know how to deal with. Too often, unbeknownst to us, unresolved pain interferes with how we function in our adult lives. It is often the case that when we experience thoughts or feelings in our adult lives that are related to emotionally distressing times in our past, (perhaps even subconsciously) we experience them with the intensity at which we felt them when they happened. So if your dad left when you were six and you never talked about it, talking about it now will bring back the feelings of a six-year-old who never cried or screamed with anger when her daddy left. Or seeing a movie with a similar theme may evoke those same intense feelings in you. Who wants to feel the fear or anger of a six-year-old as an adult? We're afraid of those feelings! We dismiss our feelings. We cover them up with substances. We deny them. Deep inside, we're still afraid no one will be there to take care of that six-year-old who did not have the developmental ability to cope with that situation alone. Don't believe me? You might in the upcoming chapters.

Professionals in the addiction field understand the connection between addiction and childhood trauma. Patrick Carnes, a renowned psychologist, has spent his entire professional career studying addiction. In the book Facing Addiction by Patrick Carnes, Ph.D., Stefanie Carnes, Ph.D. and John Bailey, M.D., the authors state, "Addicts are also likely to have experienced trauma and abuse as children. Abuse and neglect deepen distrust of others and further distort reality. Children who are neglected conclude they are not valuable. In addition, they live with a high level of anxiety because no one teaches them common life skills or provides for their basic needs. Children find ways to deaden the anxiety they inevitably feel." Addictions are the way people deaden the anxiety that lives on inside them from childhood into their adult lives.

Remember Lake Hælan? Most people tiptoe in until the feelings start. Then, scared of the feelings they experience, they run safely back to shore where they feel nothing, in their world that is bleak and brown. Safe. In their addictions.

Dr. Ablow tells us, "Confronting your pain will not paralyze you. It will allow new parts of you to be born. It is no different for those who use other pathological behaviors to anesthetize themselves. Compulsive gambling, sexual addictions, addiction to nicotine, and addiction to food are all behavioral ways that people avoid the pain that could ultimately be their path to new, healthier chapters of their lives. And what's worse, far from insulating them from suffering, these strategies actually cause their suffering to skyrocket. If you are hostage to any one of these behaviors, start thinking of it as a smoke screen that is covering up your pain and blocking your path to a better life. If you are overweight, then losing weight is only the first reward you'll get from dieting. Finding yourself is the greater reward."

Making it through Lake Hælan takes courage. "Beating an addiction requires great strength, but addiction and its psychological roots are very powerful, too," says Dr. Ablow. "That's why addicts relapse so frequently." I suspect the psychological roots he is referring to are the painful emotions addicts have stored inside for a lifetime. At some point, every one of us addicts has to choose: stay on the dreary side of the lake or harness our courage, build a support team, get into therapy, attend group meetings, do whatever you've gotta do to keep wading through the gross side of the lake to where the water reaches the very tip of the top hide of life. There, you can live fully by learning how to be your best you. The YOU that you were created to be.

CHAPTER FIVE

IS FOOD ADDICTION A THING?

It's not uncommon for a person to start "acting out," or exhibiting their experience of feeling out of control after leaving home for the first time. The first time "on your own" is a prime time for addictions to take hold. That was definitely the case for me. When I left home for college at the age of 17, my parents had recently separated. My father, a very functional alcoholic, had moved to a house a few blocks from where my parents and six children (five girls, one boy, two parents; three bedrooms and one bathroom… just sayin'!) had lived our entire lives. Dad was gone; mom was "gone," too, but in a different sense. She had found her freedom and was living it up, coming home at all hours of the night. I remember, while still in high school, having to go pick her up at a bar in the middle of the night and then having to get up to go to school the next day.

I had mixed feelings when it was time to move to college, a large university three-and-a-half hours from home. My older sister was in school at the same university, but I was never more alone in my life than I was during my freshman year. I worried constantly about my younger siblings and both of my parents. My older sister was already partying like a wild child, so I rarely saw her. I isolated myself in my dorm room. I didn't know how to cope with being alone (remember the three bedrooms and the eight people in the small house in which I was raised?). I didn't know how to talk about what was happening because we never talked about anything real in our family. Nor did we feel. So I froze. Internally, I froze. Just thinking about that time in my life, I feel tension in my body even now. It feels like I'm putting back on the thick, heavy armor, the emotional straightjacket I wore for protection and survival.

Life as a freshman in college became all about food for me. Except I wouldn't eat any. Starvation became my addiction. Yes, anorexia is classified as an eating disorder, and I had it bad. But it was also part of an addiction. Foods, calories, exercise were all I would allow myself to think about. How many calories in an egg white? How many in cottage cheese? Those were the only foods I needed to know the calories for because that was all I would allow myself to eat. How much exercise is required to burn off the calories in an egg. (Really?) Yes, that was my reality. My life was out of control. And controlling food was my way to try to have some control in my life.

John Bradshaw said, "Addictions are ways to be out of control. Addictions provide relief." I felt so out of control on the inside. My addiction, the mental and physical addiction to food and everything to do with food: the calories, the amount of exercise needed to burn the calories was my "safe" way of being out of control. It was so much more socially acceptable to be out of control with my food than say, running around campus screaming my head off, shouting, "Can anyone help me? Can anyone fix what is happening to my family? Can anyone get my father to stop drinking and move home? Can anyone please get my mother to stop behaving like a rebellious teenager? Can anyone please, please, please help me to not lose my mind?" NOT FEELING ANYTHING was achieved by my focus on food. My addiction provided me relief.

Tennie McCarty says, "Food addiction is another way in which we try to exert control over the world. Whether through overeating, purging, or restriction— i.e., starvation— we know what will happen when we eat (or starve), and we know how it will affect those around us." Tragically, I knew how my weight loss would affect those around me (my family, when I would go home for holidays). I knew no one would say anything about it. And they didn't. Not one of them.

Neither of my parents, who had either lost their vision or their own minds (clearly it was the latter) said one thing about their college-aged daughter, five feet and four inches tall, who showed up weighing less than 90 pounds. Thus, reaffirming to me that I was invisible and did not matter.

My addiction of choice changed a number of times over the years, prior to my entering outpatient treatment at the age of 28. For 11 straight years I numbed my emotional pain with food, alcohol, painkillers, men, cigarettes, rage, and work. All of my addictive behaviors and substances affected every area of my life. As for my social life: I only hung out with others who were trying as desperately as I was to NOT FEEL.

Glenn Beck, himself a recovering addict, along with Keith Ablow, co-wrote a book titled, <u>The 7 Seven Wonders That Will Change Your Life</u>. In this book, they talk about the people with whom addicts socialize:

> "Misery may love company, but denial absolutely requires it. Look around you at the people you've attracted. They reflect something inside you. Unless you're working for a charity or a rehab clinic, you won't find yourself surrounded by addicts if you aren't either an addict yourself or, at the very least, an enabler. You won't find yourself surrounded by people who keep undermining you, unless you doubt or dislike yourself. You won't find yourself surrounded by people who keep asking way too much of you, unless you think your value is determined by how much people need you. You won't find yourself surrounded by people who live superficial lives filled with material things, unless you live your life the same way. I was a self-hating addict, desperately running from my truth, and I attracted people who disliked themselves and were on the run, too. They valued me for my problems, not my capacity to overcome them. And I valued them for theirs. All of us unconsciously felt as though we needed each other to stay in numbing, escapist, self-defeating patterns of thought and behavior. It was as though we had tied our shoelaces together, yet kept wondering why we continually fell flat on our faces."

We're going to get to you in just a few minutes here so be thinking about this… who *are* the people you hang out with?

I was always afraid of, intimidated by people I thought "had it all together." The all-together people in my young adult life, when I was still hiding from myself through various addictions, were the wives of the men my husband worked with. I was never so uncomfortable as when we spent time with them, although I desperately wished I fit in with them. Tragically, I carried within myself tremendous SHAME, a hallmark of addiction. The deepest part of Lake Hælan, the most painful place in the lake where the water covers your face and you can't breathe is where you face your Shame. Shame is suffocating, and I felt suffocated and stupid and oaf-ish and paralyzed by my shame when I was with the other young wives. I felt "less than," because I knew inside what a mess I was, what a mess of a family I had come from, what horrible behaviors I had engaged in over the prior many years, and how phony I was. These were ladies. They were trim and tan and they dressed right and they were, well, better than I was. They "knew" things I didn't but should have.

I specifically remember a day when one of the "together ladies" was talking about some woman whose child's feet were peeling and chaffing. "My God!" exclaimed Mrs. Together. "Everyone knows you have to put real leather shoes on your child's feet!" Laugh, laugh, laugh. They all laughed. I died inside. My child didn't wear leather shoes. And his little feet *were* peeling. "I DIDN'T KNOW!" I shouted in my head. In my heart, I cried, "I should have known! Why didn't I know! I'm a horrible mother!" My shame pounded throughout my insides and I just wanted to hide. To numb. So I did. I probably drank too much that day.

My crowd, the people with whom I felt at ease, were the people with whom I worked. We were all in sales, one of many professions filled with needy individuals who will work themselves to the bone to win a plaque that says, "SEE! I AM SOMEBODY! I MATTER! I DID GOOD!" because on the inside, they feel empty. The trophies and victories of sales bring along a false sense of okay-ness. It makes me think of a two-year-old who successfully uses the potty chair. "LOOK MOMMY! I DID GOOD! I AM GOOD!" How very sad to be so emotionally needy and desperate as an adult. That's what addiction behaviors can do for us … they quiet the emptiness within. I hung out with those who were like myself. Together we were comfortable with our individual emptiness.

Remember Dr. Gabor's quote? "Addiction is all about lack of peace. It's all about internal unrest. It's all about disconnection from the self... a desperate emptiness." I had no idea who I was. I was running on empty and headed nowhere in particular. I just needed to keep running lest I have some unwanted alone time with myself. If that happened, I might have to look at me. And then I would feel all the things I did not want to feel. So, like our iconic Forrest Gump, I just kept running.

Until I stopped. And I only stopped because I finally dug myself into a hole so deep that if I hadn't gotten help, I'd have lost my husband and maybe my children. I didn't mind losing myself. Hell, I had done that many years ago. In order to get the help I needed, I had to create a situation that was bad enough that my husband might leave me. That got my attention.

I realize that sounds a little "off," but I wholeheartedly believe I created a huge problem to save myself. I needed to believe it was to save my family, my children, and my marriage. My deep shame prevented me from thinking I was worth saving.

Gabor Mate describes addiction as being a means to help us find ourselves, which is what I believe I did by creating a crisis and needing to save my family and my marriage. "And so there is a part of us that created a conflict precisely to lead us to ourselves. It will go to extreme measures to wake you up. It will make you suffer greatly if you don't listen to it. What else can it do? That is its purpose."

I am completely and totally grateful to be a Recovering Addict. My addiction screamed loudly to get my attention as I acted out my internal unrest in unhealthy ways. The unrest had to get bad and loud and threaten the people I loved in order to get my attention. I finally woke up long enough to seek help when I thought I would lose the man I love and the children I treasure and adore. My addiction served the purpose to get my attention. To get help. To find me. To live the life I was born to live.

AND YOU?

So how about you? Prior to reading this book did you describe yourself as a food addict? How about after reading the previous chapter and hearing how the American Society of Addiction Medicine defines addiction? And what of my favorite authors? Have they influenced your thoughts about addiction? How about my story? Who cares... what

about YOUR story?

Let's lighten things up a bit here and play a game called, *Am I A Food Addict?*.

Here's how the game goes: I ask you some questions and you either get a point FOR THE CATEGORY or you don't! Don't give yourself a point for every question. If you answer any of the questions in a category "Yes," then you get ONE POINT for the category (even if you answer all of the questions in a category "yes"). Simple! So here goes:

QUESTION CATEGORY NUMBER ONE

a. Have you ever decided how much you were going to eat before you actually ate, but ended up eating significantly more than you had intended to? YES or NO

b. Have you ever found yourself "grazing" or eating for a longer period of time than you intended to? For example, perhaps you sat down to watch a movie and said you would have a bowl of popcorn and nothing more to eat during the movie. You ate the popcorn and several other things ... YES or NO

* If you answered either question "a" OR "b" "Yes," you get one point for Question Category One. If you answered both "a" and "b" "YES," you still get just one point for Question Category One.

QUESTION CATEGORY NUMBER TWO

a. Have you ever had a persistent desire to cut down on how much you eat? YES or NO

b. Have you ever had a persistent desire to lose weight? YES or NO

c. Have you lost weight at times in the past, only to gain it back? YES or NO

* If you answered either question "a, "b," or "c" "Yes," you get one point for Question Category Two. If you answered more than one question "YES," you still get just one point for Question Category Two.

QUESTION CATEGORY NUMBER THREE

a. Have you spent a great deal of time in activities necessary to obtain food? For example, have you driven around town for however long

it took to find a donut shop with the "HOT" sign flashing (or to find the *just right food* you *had to have* at that moment)? Another example would be spending a great deal of time cooking, even though you were supposed to be tending to family, attending a child's performance, being at work, or doing some other thing that you were expected to do? YES or NO

b. Have you ever spent a great deal of time eating at one sitting? For example, spending an evening home alone with food and eating for hours while watching television (or some variation of this when you spent a great deal of time eating)? YES or NO

c. Have you ever spent a great deal of time recovering from a food hangover? For example, did you eat so much that you were sick or had to miss work or another important activity? YES or NO

* *If you answered either question "a," "b," or "c" "Yes," you get one point for Question Category Three. If you answered more than one question "YES," you still get just one point for Question Category Three.*

QUESTION CATEGORY NUMBER FOUR

a. Have you ever given up or reduced the frequency of important social, occupational or recreational activities due to food, eating or your weight? For example, have you stayed home from kids activities, work-related social events, weddings, etc. because you were ashamed of your weight or couldn't comfortably attend because of your weight? YES or NO

* *In this case, if you answered question "a" "YES," then you get a point for Question Category Four.*

QUESTION CATEGORY NUMBER FIVE

a. Have you continued to eat the wrong foods, forego exercise, and maintain excess weight in spite of knowing that one or more physical problems (high blood pressure, diabetes, sleep apnea, etc.) or psychological problems (depression, anxiety, etc.) are directly caused or worsened by your weight? YES or NO

* *In this case, if you answered question "a" "YES," then you get a point for Question Category Five.*

QUESTION CATEGORY NUMBER SIX

a. (If you have had bariatric weight loss surgery, answer this question as it relates to your life prior to having had a bariatric weight loss procedure.) As time has passed, do you find that it takes more food to achieve the desired emotional or physical effect that you used to get with less food? For example, in the past, would a single serving of ice cream have satisfied your need for emotional of physical "fullness" whereas over time you needed more and more ice cream to achieve that same emotional or physical feeling? YES or NO

In this case, if you answered question "a" "YES," then you get a point for Question Category Six.

QUESTION CATEGORY NUMBER SEVEN

a. Have you ever experienced physical or emotional withdrawal when you stopped eating a certain food or stopped overeating? YES or NO

b. Have you ever found yourself substituting an unhealthy substance or behavior when you have stopped eating a particular food or stopped overeating? YES or NO

If you answered either question "a" OR "b" "Yes," you get one point for Question Category Seven. If you answered both "a" and "b" "YES," you still get just one point for Question Category Seven.

That's it! That's the quiz! Oh… you want the Answer Key! Hold your horses. First, let me say that this quiz is NOT definitive, is NOT scientific and does NOT have the power to label or diagnose you. It's somewhat like a quiz in a Glamour magazine. It's just an indicator. These questions are based on similar criteria the medical profession used in the recent past to determine if a person met the criteria for alcohol/drug addiction. I simply changed the questions to pertain to food. There is actually a testing instrument that was developed at Yale University called the Yale Food Addiction Scale, which was developed in a similar way.

I encourage you not to get worked up, no matter what the "results" of your quiz are. This is not going to diagnose you as anything! Got it? All right then.

- Add up the CATEGORY POINTS. (NOT the points for individual questions.)
  - There are only Seven Categories, so you can't have more than seven points. If you do, you either can't add any better than I can or you are counting points for individual questions.
  - IF you got a point for THREE OR MORE CATEGORIES, it's likely you have an addiction to food.

That is, if food addiction is a real thing…

IS FOOD ADDICTION REAL?

I asked people from all over the country who have had various weight loss surgery procedures, to share their opinion about whether or not food/eating is an addiction. As you read through their responses, keep in mind what you read earlier about how the American Society of Addiction Medicine defines addiction and what other professionals say about what addiction is. These responses are not about right or wrong. They are opinions of non-professional people struggling with food and weight issues. I asked the question on social media because I wanted to know if people thought food/eating is an addiction and why?

My specific, written question was, "Do you think food/eating is an addiction? Why or why not?" The responses included the following:

- "It can be. A lot of people who are overweight eat for emotional comfort or just to fill a void."
- "Sugar is the 'other white powder,' as addicting as cocaine."
- "Yes, I do. There is both an emotional and biological effect when food is consumed. I think, without a doubt, that eating can be an addiction… one that is insanely dangerous since you don't have the option of staying away, or eliminating food."
- "Heck yeah! Why else would I hide to eat a King Size KitKat? I'm a Carboholic!"
- "Yes. If it weren't, I wouldn't want to sneak and eat and feel like it's something I have to hide."
- "Yes, because it so hard to stop. It's not just a habit. It is deep rooted addiction."

- "Yes – I believe anything that can affect your dopamine and serotonin receptors can cause addiction. We are creatures that love pleasure. The problem with food though, is you cannot go cold turkey. I think carbohydrates and sugars are the biggest culprits."

- "YES!!! I always knew I was addicted to food but I didn't truly accept it until I lost my job last year and quickly put on 20 pounds. I knew at that moment in time that I'm really, truly addicted and I'm an emotional eater."

- "Absolutely."

- "Yes. Because it is."

- "Yes. I can't explain but it goes way beyond liking food."

- "It is absolutely an addiction!!!! I know beyond a shadow of a doubt, if food was heroin--I would be on skid row! It is an absolute drug for me with real physical and mental reactions when I get a fix! I fight the urge to make poor food choices every single day!! It is a mental battle just like that of an addict! The response to the poor food choices has to be a brain reaction also! For me it is! I fight hard!!"

- "If someone can explain the overwhelming desire to put food in my mouth at any time during the day, sometimes with reason and sometimes without, and eat it with reckless abandon without even tasting anything but the first few bites, the whole time knowing I should not be doing it while I do it and trying to talk myself out of it as it is happening, as something other than addiction, have at it. I, for one, cannot explain my behavior and truly feel as though it is a force that comes from within my body, or my brain, as it may be. I have no idea what it is like to be addicted to another substance, but I imagine it to be similar in nature, and am fairly sure that if food was not available for some unknown reason, I would reach for something else. It is certainly not my intention to state that I could not learn how to control this behavior, but it is my intention to tell the truth about what it feels like when it is happening and quite frankly it often feels like an out-of-body experience. Now how's that for an answer to your question???"

- "Yes. If food is used as a coping mechanism to quell emotions, it can lead to addiction. Research has verified that sugar has the same effects on the brain as cocaine, therefore if sweets are one's 'drug of choice', addiction is quite possible."

- "Yes- I think about food constantly. It makes you feel good. It dictates a lot of life and it can't be normal to worry about eating the way we do."

- "I completely feel food is an addiction that goes unrecognized and untreated. I truly find myself binging, like my alcoholic father and I truly can't help it. I get the same guilty feelings he would get after a binge, yet unlike alcohol, I cannot live without food. I wish I could think normally about food like others do."

- "Yes, because food is a source of comfort and escape. The addictive qualities of certain foods make it addictive. The caveat is that you need food to sustain yourself. You don't NEED certain drugs, alcohol or nicotine to sustain life."

- "Not all food is addictive, but certain substances (such as sugar, and those foods that quickly turn into sugar) can be. But as with all addictions it can be managed. A good counselor and support group helps."

- "Yes, because eating certain foods produces a euphoric feeling that is addicting, causing repeated behaviors."

- "Yes, it's something that I feel withdrawal from when I can't have what I want when I want it. I crave it and it's always on my mind."

- "Absolutely, it ignites the feel good chemical serotonin, just as gambling and sex and drug addictions."

- "Any compulsive and destructive behavior can be classified as an addiction."

- An addiction!! It's a crazy, twisted, addiction! People understand alcohol, drugs, even sex addictions, but there isn't much sympathy for being addicted to food. People say things like "push your chair back, quit eating" or "just don't eat things that make you not want to stop". You can always quit smoking, quit drugging, quit gambling.... but you can't quit eating. No one would ever suggest an addict have just one drink, one cigarette, etc. It's quite different when you are addicted to something you can't cut out of your life. With most people, life's greatest memories are built around food. Family holidays with the seasonal feasts. Wonderful travels accentuated with local scents and flavors. Food is truly the architect of life. Sadly, no one has a good answer for what to do when you are addicted to the foundation of your life. The battle never ends."

This last response reminds me of what Glen Beck had to say about people not being able to understand addiction: "To anyone who can't understand addiction, think about it in terms of a diet. Anyone can lose some weight for some time— but how many people can keep those twenty pounds off forever? How many people can make the decision each and every day, at each and every meal, to eat healthy and go to the gym?"

I'm guessing you can relate to that.

There were literally only three people who responded to my question that did not think food/eating could be an addiction.

This response came from the bariatric surgeon who was the moderator in the story from Chapter One: "Nope. Addiction is all made up."

THE DEFINITIVE RESPONSE: IS FOOD AN ADDICTION?

Here's what scientific researchers say:

- "Weight disorders and overeating are increasingly labeled addictions."

    - Bannon, K.L., Hunter-Reel, D., Wilson, G.T., & Karlin, R.A. (2009). The effects of causal beliefs and binge eating on the stigmatization of obesity. *International Journal of Eating Disorders, 42,* 118-124.

- "As much as classic drugs of abuse 'highjack' the brain, accumulating evidence with food suggests a similar impact," and

- "The evidence for food's addictive properties is steadily growing," and

- "… the possibility of addiction to food is supported by animal model research and increasingly by research with humans." 4 (58)

    - Gearhardt, A., Corbin, W.R., & Brownell, K.D. (2009). Food addiction: An examination of the diagnostic criteria for dependence. *Journal of Addiction Medicine, 3,* 1-7.

- Researchers studying food addiction often emphasize underlying biology, noting the shared activation of the dopamine and opiate systems by both food and drugs of abuse.

    - Stice, E., Figlewicz, D. P., Gosnell, B. A., Levine, A. S., & Pratt, W. E. (2013). The contribution of brain reward circuits to the obesity epidemic. *Neuroscience and Biobehavioral Reviews, 37*(0), 10.1016/j. neubiorev.2012.12.001.

    - Volkow, N. D., Wang, G.-J., Tomasi, D., & Baler, R. D. (2013). Pro v Con Reviews: Is Food Addictive?: Obesity and addiction: neurobiological overlaps. Obesity Reviews : *An Official Journal of the International Association for the Study of Obesity, 14*(1), 2–18.

- "There are several regions in the brain involved in the reinforcement of both feeding and drug intake," and

- "*... sugar, as common as it is, nonetheless meets many of the criteria for a substance of abuse and may be addictive for some individuals when consumed in a 'binge-like' manner.* This conclusion is reinforced by the changes in limbic system neurochemistry that are similar for drugs and for sugar." (bold and italics added)

    - Avena, N.M., Rada P., & Hoebel, B.G. (2007). Evidence for sugar addiction: Behavioral and neurochemical effects of intermittent, excessive sugar intake. *Neuroscience and Biobehavioral Reviews, 32,* 20-39.

- "The use of certain substances, as well as the consumption of certain foods can result in changes in the opiate system. Alcohol, as well as high-fat sweets can cause the release of endogenous opioids in the brain," and

- "...results thus far have painted a consistent and increasingly compelling picture. Certain foods, with sugar being the most thoroughly studied, activate the brain in ways similar to classic drugs of abuse."

    - Gearhardt, A., Corbin, W.R., & Brownell, K.D. (2009). Food addiction: An examination of the diagnostic criteria for dependence. *Journal of Addiction Medicine,*

3, 1-7.

There are plenty of researchers who disagree that food/eating can be added to the addiction classification. They note that the evidence for food being an addictive substance is inconclusive and therefore, we cannot say that food can be addictive. To this group of people, and to anyone who has closed their mind to the possibility that food can be an addictive substance, I say this: It took the AMA until 1956 to decide alcoholism was a disease and until 2013 to recognize obesity as a disease. How long before food addiction is officially recognized by the almighty medical machine.

And so… the definitive answer to the question, "Is food/eating an addiction?" … WE DON'T KNOW! But I think it is, and so do plenty of others.

I'll end this chapter with a thanks to all of those who responded to my social media question and by providing my own simple definition of an addict (regardless of substance or behavior):

> An addict is someone who knows a substance or behavior is causing problems in his/her life, or knows the substance or behavior is making existing problems worse. They very badly want to stop using the substance or behavior because they are aware of the problems it's causing for them and for others. They have tried to quit before and have been able to stop for various periods of time. *But they cannot stop for the long haul.*

Since this book is about food, let's use food as an example for this definition of addiction.

- Food is causing problems in my life, as evidenced by:
  - being obese
  - having co-morbid medical conditions directly associated with my weight
    - high blood pressure
    - diabetes
    - sleep apnea
  - you fill in the blanks for how food/weight is causing problems in your life _____
- I know my health problems would be improved if I were to lose

weight, which I am capable of doing. I have done so several times in the past. However, no matter how often I diet, or lose weight, *I can't stop* eating the wrong things.

So… are you a food addict? If so, what's an addict to do?

CHAPTER SIX

WHAT'S AN ADDICT TO DO?

What IS an addict to do? Well, that depends on what the addict wants. Do they want *abstinence* or do they want *Recovery*? There is a difference.

ABSTINENCE (WITHOUT RECOVERY) = "DRY DRUNK"

Wait! We're not even talking about alcohol here. What's up with the "Dry Drunk" thing? Remember that addiction is a chronic disease. If you are an addict, you will always be an addict. In other words, you cannot "cure" this disease. You *can* go into remission (which is abstinence), or you can go into Recovery. Remission means you are no longer using your drug or behavior of choice. You are "clean" and "sober." You are not under the influence of your addictive substance or behavior. Your brain and your reasoning are not hijacked by the denial and delusions of your "drug." Being in total remission from addiction, not just your drug of choice, also means you have not switched from one drug or unhealthy behavior to another.

In other words, you haven't quit eating sugar and started shopping excessively. In this case, you would still be "using," having switched from one "drug" (food) to another "drug," (shopping). If you quit eating all baked goods, but start drinking alcohol to "relax," you are not in remission or recovery. You are still "using." Similarly, if you give up sugar and white flour but start meeting strangers for hook-ups in cars and hotels (no, I'm not kidding, I've seen it happen several times), you are in neither remission nor recovery. You are playing Whack-A-Mole addiction.

WHACK-A-MOLE ADDICTION

I was so proud of myself for inventing the term Whack-A-Mole Addiction. Until I learned that I didn't. I wasn't upset about that for long. I just decided there are all sorts of other creative people who must love that carnival game as much as I do. I personally think all homes should have a full, carnival-sized game of Whack-A-Mole in a room all by itself. Perhaps even a room with padded walls! Then, whenever a family member needs to work off some extra energy or process through intense emotions in a healthy way, they can go to the Mole Room and whack away. The can even scream at the top of their lungs about whatever is upsetting them. Home versions of Whack-A-Mole would also be great for the economy. Some artistic folks could make covers for the "Moles" that look like the people you wish you could Whack! Kind of like the personalized bobble-heads!

Hopefully, you understand through context clues (isn't that a great couple of words implanted in ours brain from the third or fourth grade: "context clues")… Whack-A-Mole Addiction is substituting one unhealthy substance or behavior for another. It makes sense that a person would do this. After giving up an addictive substance or behavior, people are going to need to find something to replace it. UNLESS they enter a program of Recovery.

Remember, for the addicted brain, logic does not apply. It takes some time after giving up an addiction for the brain fog to clear. Without support from people who don't "get" addiction, an addict is treading on thin ice. Withdrawal, grief and cravings often lure a person back to their drug of choice or toward an addictive substitute. That is why it is nearly impossible for people who have never struggled with an addiction to understand why the alcoholic doesn't refrain from picking up a drink, why the food addict doesn't "push away from the table," or why the shopping addict doesn't get rid of their credit cards.

For some addicts, the addiction is behavioral. For many

addicts, their drug is an emotional barrier, protecting them from unpleasant thoughts, feelings, memories, bad marriages, and stressful jobs. Giving it up can leave people emotionally raw and vulnerable to relapse without a solid system of recovery.

Keep in mind that addiction affects all areas of your life: social, emotional, spiritual, financial, and occupational. If a person stops using a substance or engaging in a behavior, there is a void, biologically and emotionally. Addictive substances or behaviors are often an "Ahhhhhh…," a stress-relief to ease the emotional burdens of life. Caring for a chronically ill family member, dealing with a Scrooge of an employer, coping with a controlling spouse, enduring an unforeseen layoff, being a single parent, being in school while working a full time job, or dealing with health problems are examples of reasons we seek an emotional relief. There's nothing wrong with having a glass of wine now and then (if you're not an alcoholic or an addict of most any sort). There's nothing wrong with getting lost in a television program for a few hours now and then. Unless it interferes with being a responsible adult. There's nothing wrong with a decadent dessert now and then (if you're not an addict). You get the idea. We need to unwind. We need to develop healthy ways of doing so that do not turn into addictions themselves and again leave us neglecting loved ones, work, other areas of our lives and most importantly, ourselves.

Addicts who opt for abstinence without Recovery, who live without the chemical or behavioral means to emotional relief, are vulnerable to relapse due to the stress, the worry, the fear, and the genuine emotions associated with life's difficulties. It's not likely the addict knows healthy tools for expressing their feelings or they would have been using those instead of their chemical/behavioral escape. Even if they have knowledge of healthy coping skills, the "addiction fog" in one's brain may prevent them from utilizing healthy ways to deal with stress.

What does the person who gives up the addiction do with the life frenzy that has been relieved by a glass of wine, a box of cookies, a half gallon of ice cream, a cigarette, a joint, a pizza, a benzo, a roll in the hay (not real hay, like for horses… *you know*). Without their "drug," no unhealthy drug substitute, and no program of recovery, what happens?

Well, I've heard tell (note the intended secretive, "gossipy" tone connoted in those few words?), addicts without their drug have been known to have temper tantrums and nasty attacks of taking feelings out in ugly ways on unsuspecting creatures like spouses, children, grocery store clerks, dogs, bank tellers, phone solicitors, cats, and many an anonymous driver. Or major grief and depression set in and the abstinent addict isolates from others. They may maintain the bare minimum required to get by, but the people in their lives see that something is wrong. Whether angry, isolated or "getting by," the abstinent addict continues to negatively affect the lives of those around them. They also miss out on living life fully. And they are doing nothing to heal the relationship with themselves.

The addicts' feelings are going to come out if chemical or behavioral blankets are not masking them. Our addictions often serve to harness the emotions we don't know how to deal with in healthy, appropriate ways. People who are abstinent (clean/sober) but not in Recovery become overwhelmed with raw emotions. Some describe the unleashing of previously "medicated" emotions as, "I felt like I was losing my mind." Others experience a tremendous amount of physical energy (because that is what emotions are – energy). Others, who may have been using their addiction to feel *something, anything,* because they are depressed, fall into despair without their drug. They "shut down," struggling to make it through the day.

Abstinence alone frequently leaves a person emotionally fragile, depending on what other "issues" they have. A majority of patients who have bariatric surgery carry quite a bit of emotional baggage that needs to be shed, along with the excess pounds. For persons who have had no pre-surgical education about the emotional and psychological changes that take place following surgery, I say it's like we sent them into the operating room, cut their arms and legs off, then sent them home and told them to swim.

People can be at such a loss without the comfort, security and "Ahhhhh…." that food provided. I had a lady tell me the day she went home from the hospital following her bariatric procedure, she literally stood at her refrigerator and ate, knowing she could do great harm to her pouch. Another woman, following surgery, bought bag after bag of Nacho Cheese Doritos and licked the flavoring off them. Although she didn't do her body any physical harm, she spent a considerable amount of time (away from her job? her kids? her partner?) sitting and licking cheese-flavored salt off of chips. She spent emotional energy, stating she felt "weak" and "pathetic" sitting by herself licking artificial flavoring off chips and throwing them away. The shame of addiction was very much alive in her heart and mind.

A good friend of mine is a bariatric surgeon. He "gets" the addiction piece and he and his wife, a bariatric nurse and program manager, provide more psychological pre- and post-operative support to their patients than any other practice I've seen. My friend was distraught after one of his patients died (the *only* one of his patients who has passed away in the short run after having surgery). My friend, while searching his mind, feared he had somehow missed something in the man's medical history. He then told me that a family member of the man who passed came to let the surgeon know that the man caused his own death. The day after returning home from having his bariatric surgery, the man went to a pub and ate and drank "just as he always did – too much." The man who died had not indicated to his doctor prior to surgery that he drank on a regular basis. He was addicted to alcohol and food. His addictions killed him.

Addictions kill a lot more people than death certificates would indicate. Actually, there probably isn't a single death certificate that reads, "Cause of death: Addiction." I can't even begin to fathom the actual number of deaths directly related to addiction. Think of how many death certificates claim diabetes, heart attacks, strokes, or sleep apnea when the actual cause of death was addiction to food. How many deaths from "lung cancer" are really due to addiction to nicotine? Many a person who is killed in an automobile accident, in an "accidental" drowning, by an "accidental" overdose, or in a domestic violence incident are really victims of alcohol/other drug addiction.

Abstinence means getting rid of the addictive substance. Period. For some (very few) people, they get rid of the addictive substance or behavior, carry on and *seem* to do all right in life. I am skeptical, however, when I hear stories about people just stopping any addictive behavior cold turkey and reportedly "doing just fine." In my many years of experience, there are few people who suffer with addictive substances/behaviors who don't have *some* underlying issues. I've been wrong before, and it may be true that for a certain percentage of people, simply being rid of the substance is all they need to do in order to live a productive life.

A "Dry Drunk," then, is being abstinent from the addictive substance or behavior. Period. Any underlying issues likely go unaddressed. Any "isms" related to addiction go merrily along. The "isms" of addiction, you ask? Although not all addictions end in "ism," the "isms" are discussed openly in the Recovery community. In fact, one of the first books I had in mind to write was to be titled, The "Ism's" of Alcohol. I may still write it one day. Who knows?

If you know people who are addicts, particularly if their lives intersect with yours in meaningful ways, then you have experienced the "isms" firsthand. Mind you, as you read on, that I am NOT saying that addicts are bad people. In fact, quite the contrary (remember who's writing this)! Addicts are, for the most part, really great people like all other people. They suffer from a disease. A chronic disease, which, like other diseases, such as Type 2 Diabetes, COPD, Rheumatoid Arthritis, some cancers, and a number of others, cannot be "cured," but can go into remission.

Human behaviors are not always so great but I, at least, believe people come into the world "good" and most would like to do "good" in the world. The behaviors of people in active addiction are not always what the majority would refer to as "good." Behaviors such as stealing possessions and money to buy drugs, leaving children alone to drink and party with friends, neglecting loved ones to spend time alone with food, using household money for gambling, using corporate credit cards to pay for unauthorized purchases, staying at work all hours of the night to avoid being at home, staying on pornography sites for hours at a time after promising your spouse you would stay away from them completely, sneaking and lying about the food you eat while heading to the gym with your significant other, or buying yourself the 150th pair of shoes when your kids need art supplies, dance shoes or athletic equipment. These are all probably really good people engaging in really selfish, addictive behaviors.

Speaking of selfish, it may be the number one "ism" of addicts. The unspoken motto of an addict is, "I want what I want when I want it," often with the spoken or silent footnote, "and the hell with anybody else."

I knew I was being selfish when I left my young husband home with our three very young children way too often. But the voice of my addiction was more powerful: "You deserve a job where you have friends and reminders that you are good at what you do." The inside voice of shame and insecurity that I didn't want to face spoke to me, as well: "You don't know how to be a mother. Your love isn't enough. You aren't enough. You don't know how to love other people. You're not lovable yourself." My need to run away from my fears, from my insecurity, from my shame and from myself showed in behaviors that looked very selfish, and were very selfish.

Addicts have a difficult time with this. Most of us don't think of ourselves as being "selfish." In fact, particularly in my work with men and women dealing with the horrors of obesity, I hear, "I give and give to others all the time," "There's almost nothing I wouldn't do for someone else," and "I take care of everyone else and neglect myself." Remember my examples of "surface responses" from a previous chapter? These are examples of what I refer to as "surface responses," or the things we say about ourselves, which are not false, but only represent part of the whole picture.

I'll finish this example, but will first give you an example of a partial truth surface response that I used for a long time until someone who knows me well and cared about me shared honest feedback that clarified the issue. I can have a colorful "potty mouth." I was raised in an environment in which not only my parents, but all adults I knew spewed "shit," "hell" and "damn" as regularly as words such as "the," "it," and "and." I also spew "shit," "hell" and "damn" in a similar manner, adding words I learned in college, too! (The only arena in which I am 98% potty-mouth free is around my grandchildren, although I have slipped up a time or two. My kids thought it would be me who corrupted their innocents with my language, but as it turns out, it's the LOVEBUG who fails to monitor his Midwestern vernacular around the babies. The SAME Lovebug who, along with this co-worker, mentioned to me his discomfort related to my trifecta of filthy words when speaking to patient groups.) My typical retort, my "surface response," was, "That's just who I am." My co-worker, without missing a beat, replied, "You don't have to be."

Ouch. She was absolutely right. I didn't have to be. So why did I? What did I need or want by using those words in my professional life? I had always chalked my use of swear words up to a habit I continued from what I learned as a child. My "potty mouth" was "just part of who I am," I said. Well, I had also grown up in a world of smokers and drinkers. I followed through with both of those behaviors, as well. And stopped them because those things were not things with which I wanted to be identified. The "potty mouth?" It never bothered me. But saying, "it's just who I am," was an easy answer.

As I gave it some thought, I allowed for there being truth to my use of profanity being a "habit" that "I learned." Yet, I had to look deeper, as I ask others to do. What did I need or want from holding on to a habit that is offensive to some people? What did I gain from using language that certainly isn't necessary, particularly when in professional settings? I realized that I wanted acceptance. In addition, I wanted to be considered "relatable." I thought people would be less intimidated by my "title" if I were down to earth with my language. I wanted patients to see me as just an ordinary person who has struggled in many of the same ways they have. Wake-up call! I can do that without including words that people may take offense to. I can show respect for others and for myself, and for the fact I worked very hard to obtain a PhD while remaining down-to-earth. I have experienced many of the same struggles as the people I treat and I have used the same tools to work through my issues that I am offering to others. Using profanity is, and was, a choice for me. It has proven to be a way to lose the respect of a percentage of people in any group.

Back to the people who give the surface response that they constantly take care of others, but fail to take care of themselves. By the way, many of these people are often angry because "others don't reciprocate." I typically acknowledge that it's very likely the case that "caregiving" is a large part of the person's character and note they likely learned to be a giving person throughout their life. When asked to look more deeply at what needs they get met by being available to others and doing for others, people recognize needing "to be liked," "to be appreciated," "to be part of the group," and "to feel valued."

Am I a selfish person? Are these others selfish people? Or are we sick people who need to get well? Are we using what we know to get what we need? Or is there some of it all at play?

Let's look at some other situations.

Sometimes addicts need to be taken care of. An alcoholic sometimes needs help to get off the floor and into bed. An addict may need to be taken to the hospital after an overdose. A food addict may need a person to physically care for them, to include getting them food, as they are too obese to get out of bed. A gambling addict may need to be bailed out of debt. Selfish? Sick? Both?

There is no shame in being an addict. People don't choose to be addicts. And yet many choose not to get help for their addiction.

The selfish behaviors of an addict are associated with the biological disease of addiction that affects the brain, with the underlying emotional issues a person is running from and the relief they are seeking from their addiction. The selfish behaviors of addicts are inextricably entwined with the shame that burns constantly within the addict. The behaviors of an addict *are* very often selfish from an external perspective. Internally, the addict is drowning in shame and staying afloat with defenses. Their behaviors appear selfish. Their motive is survival.

I personally want to call it selfish when a person becomes aware of their reality, of their addiction, and chooses not to get help for it. I don't mean to judge, and realize I have no way of knowing the depth of a person's pain, trauma, loss or grief. Nor do I have insight into the strength of another's character or spirit, their level of intelligence, education or resiliency. Therefore, I can only say that, like an addict's behavior, their decision to put forth the effort into being in Recovery, is not mine to judge. Many of the behaviors of an addict, as well as a conscious decision not to seek Recovery, do *appear* to be selfish.

Selfishness, nonetheless, is one of the "isms" of addicts. Isms are behaviors and attitudes that many addicts display. Addicts can be notoriously controlling, manipulating persons and situations in order to get what they want. "Controlling" is really just another way of saying manipulative, by the way. People don't like thinking of themselves as being manipulative, but all of us are to some extent. Letting one's ego (another "*ism*") get in the way of making sound, healthy decisions is another common denominator of addicts. Defensiveness strategies are also isms. I will address these isms in more detail in a later chapter. For now, understand that these "isms" are based on fear, are fueled by shame, are an attempt to get needs met in unhealthy ways, and are common to most addicts.

Simply being without the drug of choice does not automatically eradicate the isms associated with addicts' behaviors or attitudes. Abstinence from a drug or addictive behavior leaves an addict in physical or emotional withdrawal, complete with a set of behaviors and attitudes (the isms) formerly used to get the addict what he/she wanted when he/she wanted them, no matter what. In recovery circles, they often say, "a Dry Drunk is a sober a*%hole."

Abstinence/sobriety, is not a pleasant place to live. It's like hanging out in the murkiness of Lake H, without the drug to anesthetize you from the pain you are wallowing in, and being miserable indefinitely.

RECOVERY

Recovery is so much more than abstinence. Addiction is a disease. It is a chronic disease and so, like other chronic diseases, addiction can go into remission. Remission, when speaking of addiction, is the equivalent of abstinence. If you are an addict it is only when you are not engaging in an addictive behavior or using an addictive substance that you are in remission from addiction.

Take me, for example. I played Whack-A-Mole addiction for many years. I started with food, then, when my life was literally in danger (think Karen Carpenter), I started drinking. Alcohol kept me away from myself (my sadness, my hurt, my feelings, my thoughts), which is exactly where I wanted to be. Out of touch with emotions. Over the next several years, I randomly hit the Narcotics Mole, the Men Mole, the Nicotine Mole, the Alcohol Mole, the Narcotics Mole and the Work Mole. Not once was I in remission from my disease of addiction. And I was nowhere close to being in Recovery.

Not until I was in enough emotional pain was I ready to look at the reality that I am an addict. My drug of choice changed over time and was not limited to one substance or behavior. It was anything that I engaged in to avoid me. My addiction continued as long as I participated in ways to avoid myself. My addictions led in the direction of the destruction of my self-esteem, my marriage, my family, my soul.

When my marriage was at a breaking point, I knew I had to face whatever I needed to face or lose my family and continue on a path of insanity, running from one thing to another in vain attempts to fill an inner emptiness. Two things were necessary for me to become whole, to be both abstinent (in remission) and to live in Recovery from my disease. I had to stop using substances, behavior and people as "drugs." No one can be in recovery (or remission) from addiction if they continue to use. You can't be dry if you're still swimming in a swimming pool. It's impossible.

To be in Recovery from my addictions I needed to learn to love myself. I needed to heal from the inside. No one could do it for me. Yet, I couldn't do it alone. Others could be there to support me, to guide me, and to assist me, but no one could do the work of healing my inner hurts but me. No one but me could fix what I had been hiding from and running from through all of my addictions.

And so, I began the journey of Recovering from Addiction. Recovery, for me, has been the process of learning to love myself, learning to have compassion for myself, learning to hold myself accountable, learning to treat myself with respect, and learning to be able to truly love others. Recovery is a way of life. It's learning things about how to deal with life in healthy ways. It's learning to recognize your feelings and how to express them appropriately. We all grew up learning what we lived in our homes, our neighborhoods, our schools. That is true for our parents and their parents and their parents. So there's no blame-game to play. It's just a fact. Kids learn from those around them. When we grow up, we live what we learned. Until, and if, we learn new ways, we will continue to live out what we learned in our childhoods. That includes attitudes and behaviors.

In my home, there was a lot of anger accompanied by a lot of yelling. Followed by tense periods of the silent treatment. Fortunately, there was also plenty of laughter and playfulness at times.

Guess how I behaved in my marriage? With a lot of yelling, silent treatments, and enough playfulness to *almost* create a balance between the yuck and the fun. I never learned at home or from extended family to talk through conflict, to give and take, or to be able to be wrong and say, "I'm sorry" or "I love you."

I needed the help of other people who understood that addictions are an impossible way to try to fix a biological crossing of wires. Addictions are an impossible way to outrun pain that has been held inside, but that comes out in ways that often hurts ones self and others. For me, some of those others included people in recovery from their own addictions, who had walked the path of Recovery ahead of me. They reached out to me and shared the many tools they had been taught that helped them fight cravings, deal with stress in healthy ways, set boundaries with others, and work through painful feelings.

As I learned about the process of Recovery, I also had what seemed like incessant therapy. I had therapy in the outpatient treatment program. When that was over, I had aftercare counseling every week for a year and then "as needed" for several years after that. My husband and I also went to couples counseling AND to a couple's group. In addition to that, I attended 12 Step meetings. Sound excessive? It wasn't. In the first two to three years after giving up my security blankets, my adult pacifiers, my addictions, I started to grow up.

I learned that my feelings would not kill me. I (started) to learn that I could express anger without screaming (and scaring my children in the process). I was shown how to have a discussion with my husband without being critical or completely defensive. I learned that I had value as a person, that I wasn't invisible, or unintelligent, and that I mattered.

We immersed ourselves in the learning process, in the Recovery Process. And we were willing to go in debt to pay for it all. Hence, I have little tolerance for people who might be financially strapped but *could* make therapy work in their budget, but won't go to therapy or do whatever it is that they have to do to get healthy and get happier. Many of these same people are willing to pay for cigarettes or the fanciest cell phone or the most extravagant cable package.

There's no way out but through. If you aren't willing to put forth the effort, whatever it takes, you may be abstinent, but you will not know the joys of living in Recovery from Addiction. That's the colorful side of Lake Hælan.

I'll share one story, the story that ultimately led me to doing what I'm doing today. After a year or so of completing the outpatient treatment program, I knew I wanted to work in some way in the field of addiction and recovery. I envisioned doing marketing for a treatment center or something along those lines. I was planning to get back into school and was studying for an exam required to get into a Master's program.

Part of the sacrifice the Lovebug and I made so that we could rebuild our marriage and nurture our family was to sell our house. We had to sell our house and purchase a less expensive one, in part because we were paying for treatment and the plethora of therapies. A greater reason was that I quit the job I had selling encyclopedias. I made good money doing that. The problem was twofold. As I mentioned earlier, sales was an unhealthy way for me to feel ok about myself. Secondly, I would work countless hours, at the expense of spending time with my family so I could win a sales contest and get a cheap plaque or trophy that confirmed to me that I had value. I traveled out of town with co-workers who, like me, were big partiers. My job was part of my addiction.

Recovery requires letting go of people and places that are threats to your sobriety. I was willing to do whatever it took to find and love *me* and create the life I wanted with my husband and family. I did get another job, although I was miserable doing it. Since sales was my only work experience since graduating from college, aside from bartending, which was clearly out of the question, I got a job selling commercial time for a local television affiliate. I didn't watch TV and had no interest in what I was doing. But it was income.

When I quit the encyclopedia sales job, we incurred more debt paying for our healthy new life, and we needed a lower mortgage. We sold our home and, as a side note, were led to live next door to one of my very best friends in life to this day. I loved the life we were building as I got sober and entered a full program of Recovery. I had never had true girlfriends before. Of course not. I didn't like myself and I had carried so much shame inside, it was impossible to believe anyone else would accept me. I had plenty of "surface" friends, but when I stopped working, I realized how equally yoked those women and I had been. They were empty people, searching for some way – any way – to feel better about themselves, like I was. I had to leave those friends and those playgrounds and find healthier people and places to play.

In the process of treatment, aftercare, 12 Step meetings and couples group, we started making couples friends, people who were also putting forth tremendous efforts to let go of addictions, find and love themselves, and build healthier lives. In that process, I made another amazing friend I still turn to when I need support, guidance, feedback and unconditional love. She is my "soul sister."

One night, late in the night, I sat studying at our dining room table. One of my precious little twin daughters, who was three or four years old at the time, came toddling down the stairs in her purple footie pj's with her tattered blue blankie, LeeLee, trailing at her side. In her sleepy, sweet baby girl voice, she squeaked, "Will you rock me?" It's likely that in the past, I wouldn't have had time for any such thing. I would have sent her back up to bed and tended to what I wanted to do. Not now. Now I knew the importance of taking time for my babies, particularly when they were asking for it. "Of course!" I happily replied.

As I rocked that tiny, precious, innocent daughter of mine, I was filled beyond capacity with joy that overflowed in the form of tears onto her fine, thin baby hair. My thought was, "In this moment, I am experiencing the kind of joy that I believe few people experience in a lifetime." I knew I had to encourage, guide, help, hold the hands of, and teach others who wanted to know the full, colorful, joy-filled side of life, people who were willing to get through the dark, scary, dank side of Lake Hælan to the beautiful side.

Recovery. It's living fully. It's a mindset that says, "This is the kind of person I want to be. In order to become that person, I will ask, with every decision I have to make, 'Will doing this move me closer to being the person I want to be or farther from it?'" Simple. NOT EASY. But worth striving for.

Recovery is a determination. It is a commitment to putting forth effort every single day to move, if even an inch, in the direction toward where you want to be.

Recovery is a process. It is not an event. It's not a quick fix. It's living in the present and staying focused on the moment. Enjoying the moment. Knowing that "in this moment, things are ok."

Recovery is an attitude. It's being open-minded to learning things about yourself that are painful at first, but help you become your best self. It's a willingness to listen to others who have information you need. It's saying "yes" to possibilities.

Recovery is the process of learning to live life as a healthy adult who loves oneself and is therefore better able to love others.

Let me hold your hand and give you some tips about how to get from the dark side of the lake to the point where shame covers your entire being so you can begin to walk peacefully, joyfully, into the crystal clear water and onto the beautiful, lush side of the lake where *you* can learn to love yourself and to live fully!

CHAPTER SEVEN

DO WHAT YOU'RE TOLD

Who wants to be told what to do? I'd have to respond, "It depends on the circumstances." If I'm driving, I don't want a "back seat driver" telling me what to do every five minutes. If I've landed myself in a ditch, I definitely want someone who knows how to navigate the vehicle out of the ditch telling me exactly what to do!

Addiction eventually lands people in "ditches" of sorts. Maybe your food addiction led to the "ditch" of acute medical problems. Perhaps your food addiction interfered in your marriage to the point your spouse was ready to call it quits. Maybe binges that lasted throughout the night resulted in too many days of missing work and you were fired.

People in ditches need others to tell them how to get out. And to help them once they're out.

In Recovery circles, these "ditches" are better known as "hitting rock bottom." Some people talk about having a "high bottom" while others speak of having "low bottoms." I think one day I'll write a book and call it "My High Bottom." That's got a clever ring to it! It'll be about how, relative to many other addicts, my "hitting rock bottom" appeared to have fewer, less drastic consequences. People with "low bottoms" share stories of having lost custody of their children as a consequence of their addiction. They have been in jail or prison (perhaps repeatedly) due to their addiction and/or behaviors while "high." "Low bottoms" include losing jobs, marriages, friends, family members, and money as a direct result of addiction and associated behaviors. The lowest of "low bottoms" are situations in which a person has taken the life of another in a drunk driving accident, while committing armed robbery when under the influence, or by falling asleep with a lit cigarette and burning the house down. Or they kill themselves.

I had a "high bottom." I hadn't lost my family. Yet. I hadn't lost my job. Yet. I hadn't physically harmed anyone. Yet. I hadn't gotten in any legal trouble. Yet.

I could have. But for the grace of my Unseen Protector, I did not lose my family, I did not lose my job, I did not physically harm anyone and I did not incur legal problems. However, if I had kept using, I would have. Or I may have died myself.

My bottom was the threat of losing my husband and my children. I knew that if I did not seek treatment for my addiction, I would have lost my family. I had to give up my addictive behaviors or risk losing everything. When the pain of living in active addiction became more painful than facing myself, my reality, my pain, and my addiction, I took the steps and walked through the dark side of the lake to the sparkling waters that represent Recovery.

Prior to entering the outpatient treatment program, I sought counseling. I sensed my husband's increasing impatience with my job and frequent absences from home. I realized I was running out of excuses to give my doctor needing more narcotic pain medication. I knew the doo doo was about to hit the fan.

It amazes me when I think back about the course of events that unfolded from there. That invisible Guiding Force led me where I needed to be.

I called the local Community Mental Health Center and scheduled an appointment to see a therapist.

Upon meeting my new therapist, I knew I was in the wrong place. I had been in therapy before, and could tell a seasoned therapist from a novice. The poor young woman I met when I entered her office at the Community Mental Health Center that day didn't even need to open her mouth before I knew ours was not a match made in patient-client heaven. I was a mere 28 years of age at the time, and I think she was maybe all of 24. She timidly asked me questions from the Counseling 101 textbook and I impatiently answered her. Although I really just wanted to get up and walk out, I did not do so. That 50-minute session couldn't get over quickly enough. I remember nothing about it except I knew I was not going to get the help I needed from the lovely, yet inexperienced "therapist," Pollyanna. (Yes, I know I that's rude. Yet, that was exactly my mindset at the time.)

Upon leaving, I called the Community Mental Health Center I had just exited, and told the woman who answered that I needed help, but the person I had seen was not the counselor I needed. Could they schedule me with someone else? Please. She informed me that someone would get back to me.

Someone did. His name was Director of the Community Mental Health Center. He was also a therapist. Mr. Director-Therapist informed me, "We have confidence in all of our providers." He asked my reasons for wanting to see someone other than Pollyanna. Rather than quipping, "Because *I'm* even old enough to be her mother," I told him the truth. "I don't think she's going to be able to help me." Who knows what else I said, but his response was, "All right, then. I'll see you for therapy."

Oh, crap! I wasn't certain I wanted Mr. Director-*and*-Therapist to see me! I could tell even on the phone that *he* probably *could* help me! That frightened me as much as Pollyanna *not* being able to help me! I am so very grateful I had the courage to speak up for myself that day. Doing so landed my addicted young self in that man's office. Exactly where I needed to be.

He was definitely a wise one, this guy! Almost immediately, he started asking questions about the family in which I was raised, my "family of origin."

"What is it with these counselor types?" I wondered to myself, wanting so badly to bolt out of his office. "They're always wanting to talk about the family I grew up in. My problems now have nothing to do with them."

When I had attended counseling in college, any time the therapist started discussing the "family of origin," I quit going to counseling. THAT was one topic I was not willing to discuss. Translation: I was not yet ready or willing to acknowledge or experience my feelings about my family members or my childhood. I was too afraid.

However, when Mr. Director-Therapist asked about my family of origin, I knew that if I wanted to get help, I would need to cooperate. And I trusted him for some reason. I told him about the events leading up to my departure for college, about my father's drinking, my mother's return to teenagerdom, and about my acute loneliness. I filled him in on the anorexia/food addiction and shared how drinking had gotten me through school. He listened and didn't judge or scold me.

Shortly before the end of our third or fourth session, he asked, in a way suggesting his question was a mere afterthought, "Could *you* be an alcoholic?" Stunned, I thought about the drinkers I knew, comparing myself to them. I certainly didn't drink like my father did, and he was an alcoholic. I knew I didn't drink as much as my older cousins or my aunts or uncles. One aunt had already died from her alcoholism. Another was barely hanging on to the party life with her skinny, frail body with the bloated belly. I didn't seem to be anything like they were. Not wanting to appear defensive and respond immediately, I told him I would consult with my spouse and let him know at my next session.

Steve was just as baffled as I. "How could *you* be an alcoholic?" he asked, the confusion about the mere possibility of such a thing evident in his voice. "You hardly ever drink anymore." That was true. After getting married, and especially after having the kids, I didn't drink very often.

I only drank when I was out of town with those low-down co-workers of mine who were such a terrible influence on me (!!!). Steve didn't know that when I was on those work trips, we drank A LOT. The fact that I lacked an off switch was apparent to everyone, even though few of them seemed to have an off switch themselves.

The other thing my trusting (naïve) young husband didn't know was that I was taking prescription medication with codeine in it every day. He thought I took them only when I had a migraine. I wasn't about to tell him the truth. Nor was I going to enlighten Mr. Director-Therapist man about that matter. I wanted help (to save my marriage and family). I never said I wanted to quit taking codeine. And I was only asked to discuss whether or not I might be an alcoholic. He hadn't said anything about *quitting* drinking, nor had he asked me about pills.

"No," I told the Director at the time of my next visit. "Steve doesn't think I'm an alcoholic and neither do I." After explaining to him our joint marital assessment of my alcohol consumption patterns, I informed the Director-Therapist that I wasn't getting the help I needed quickly enough. These weekly sessions were simply not providing me with the answers to my questions. Therapy was not offering solutions to my problems in a timeframe consistent with my expectations. Oh, how I chuckle looking back at myself!

Ah, this experienced man wasn't fooled for a minute by the likes of me. In fact, I'd say he got one over on me! "I have an idea about a place you could go for answers and get them more quickly." He explained that right there in our little Midwestern town was a place I could go to therapy five nights a week for four hours each evening. It was a program for people who had grown up in alcoholic homes or who were living with alcoholics. I would be finished with the program in six short weeks. Not exactly what I wanted to do for six weeks, but I knew I still didn't have the answers to my questions and this once-a-week thing wasn't cutting it. The question I wanted answered in therapy, by the way, was, "Should I stay in my marriage?" No one knew that but me. Whether or not I was an alcoholic or addict was as far from my mind as the Earth is from Pluto. I just wanted to know if I should stay or if I should go.

"Okay," I reluctantly agreed. "I'll go to this program. But it'll have to wait about three months. There's this sales contest that I really want to win. When it's over, I'll go."

I suspect Mr. Director-Therapist never expected to see me again.

Oh, how very internally desperate I was for external validation that I was an okay person. I needed to win a sales contest to give me a false sense of importance before I could worry about my marriage, my family, my children, my SELF. That, my friends, is the insanity of addiction. Truly messed up priorities and undoubtedly clouded judgment.

True to my word, after winning the sales contest that reassured me I was worthwhile, I called the Community Mental Health Center and asked for a referral to the program for persons raised in alcoholic homes. He hadn't told me that was only one track at the treatment center. There was also a program for the alcoholics and addicts.

OUTPATIENT TREATMENT

I observed the evenings' proceedings for about three nights before uttering a word. On the fourth day, I asked to speak to my small group counselor. There were approximately 30 people in the program; we were divided into two groups for "small group," which took up about half of every evening. Julie, a thin, attractive woman in her late 40's, listened to me attentively, as I shared, "I don't think this is the place for me." She said nothing, so I continued, "The people here... they, they... well, they've had really rough lives. There are people out there who have been in jail! Others were locked in closets when they were little! Or beaten! I had a great childhood! I had a nice home. And a family. And I don't have anything in common with these people!" I believe my voice had a pleading quality to it, implying, "Please! Get me out of here! I'm different than these people. I'm better than these people! I do not belong in a program with these people!" Without changing her serene expression, Julie simply said to me, "Keep coming back. And trust the process."

What the hell did that mean? Trust the process. I just wanted to quit! But no one had told me yet if I should stay in my marriage or if I should leave. So I chose to endure more time with my fellow inmates... I mean, treatment participants.

That same evening, as I was stewing over Julie's words, "'Keep coming back,' and 'Trust the process,'" something happened that struck a chord deep within my head, or my psyche, and in my soul. A woman in "small group," where people processed their individual homework assignments, read aloud a letter she had written to her father. In my mind, my father had always been a hero of sorts to me. In spite of his drinking, he and I had a close bond when I was a child. My dad always told me I was "different" than "those Kelly women" (the females on my mother's side of the family). He said I was "special." I was his "buddy" when I was a young child, always running from the garage to the kitchen to fetch him a beer. I helped him as he worked on his cars by handing him tools and hanging out with him. I did not want to hear anything bad about my father and I was certainly never going to say anything bad about him.

By the time the woman in small group stopped reading her letter, I, who hadn't cried in years, was literally curled up in a fetal position on the floor sobbing. I haven't the foggiest idea what she had written, but it resonated with something deep inside me.

I kept coming back. I started to trust the process.

The counselors at this place were wise, like Mr. Therapist-Director. I couldn't pull anything over on them, either! In spite of dutifully completing my homework every night, sharing with my group members, and doing what I thought was a darn good job in my program, I was singled out one evening and asked to go with JoAnn. She wanted to ask me some questions.

I wasn't sure exactly who JoAnn was, but I knew she worked for the treatment center in some official sort of capacity. Without letting me know why, she started asking me all sorts of questions. I answered her questions honestly. They were about my own use of alcohol and drugs. Steve and I had decided together that I wasn't an alcoholic, so I wasn't worried about failing her questionnaire. I had never even tried any "real drugs," with the exception of marijuana a few times when I was in college. I hated that stuff. It just made me laugh. Really hard. Out loud. I was always embarrassed and would go into the bathroom and laugh, out loud, by myself. I was sure using marijuana five times did not a drug addict make. So I wasn't worried about her drug questions, either. Although I *was* a bit nervous about what she might have to say about the codeine. Yet I answered her questions about pain medications honestly, as well.

"Well, no wonder!" she said aloud. "No wonder what?" I asked, also aloud. She sounded somewhat gleeful to me as she announced, "No wonder things aren't adding up. You're not only the family member of an alcoholic, you're an alcoholic and drug addict yourself!"

I'm certain I looked around the 6x6 closet-like room to find the other person JoAnn was speaking to. I knew without a doubt it wasn't me she was referring to as an alcoholic and a *drug addict*!

I was shocked and indignant. "A *drug addict?*" She had lost all credibility with me! I spewed, "I was given some drugs wrapped in aluminum foil after a Bee Gees concert when I was in college. One of the band members gave it to me. I didn't even know what it was! I gave it to my sister!" Obviously, I had forgotten my prior concern about the codeine, as those two words, drug addict, did not include prescription medication in my mind. Drug addict meant things like pot and hash and cocaine. Cocaine! "JoAnn," I implored. "My sister and her friends used to use my makeup mirror for lines of coke. I would come home from work at the bar and there they'd be, in our apartment, in my bedroom with my makeup mirror, with lines of cocaine. I would leave the house! I never once even tried it!" (I think I knew intuitively that if I did ever try it, there would be no turning back for me.) I fessed up about the Black Beauty. "I did try a Black Beauty one time but I could feel my heart beating out of my chest." I held my hand four inches from my chest, indicating how hard my heart beat when I took that speed. I then remembered the "white cross" I took every night when I worked late at the bar. It pepped me up.

"And," I added earnestly, "I could have answered some of those questions about alcohol either way. I mean...," my pitch rising and my tone increasingly hysterical. "But you didn't," JoAnn stated directly and emphatically. "You didn't answer them differently."

The rest of that meeting is a blur. How could I be an alcoholic? Didn't all of those people in college drink as much as I did? Maybe even more? And didn't it matter that I rarely ever drank now? How can you be an alcoholic if you don't drink very often? How can a person be a drug addict if they have only ever tried one or two... or three drugs? I didn't *need* alcohol or drugs to survive. I wouldn't have physical withdrawals without alcohol or any drug.

By the end of the night, I had been switched from the program for family members to the program for the alcoholics and addicts. And I had dumped all of the codeine I possessed down the toilet at the treatment center.

I was scared. I was also more relieved than I have ever been in my life. It fit. Deep inside, I knew it was true. I was an alcoholic. I was a drug addict.

Steve started the program for family members. Our six weeks began anew.

And that is where my life started. I had a high bottom. I am so very grateful for that. Whatever kind of bottom you have if you're an addict, help IS available! Seek it!

What about you? How far down has your bottom gotten? (I know you're making a joke in your mind about your rear end right now!) How bad are your health conditions because of your weight? Has your love affair with food (your primary relationship) interfered in your relationships with loved ones? Do you miss your children's school events because you would rather stay home alone and binge? Are you too ashamed of the way you look to be seen at their games, concerts or plays? Do you worry about your family members being embarrassed by your size so you avoid their activities? Have you stolen food? Do you lie about how many people you are buying food for when you go to the drive thru? Is your productivity at work less because you are thinking about food or eating food when you should be working? Have you lost a job due to your addiction? Is your life in physical danger because of your addiction? Have you lost respect for yourself because of your addiction and related behaviors? Have you lost hope because of your food addiction? How low is your bottom headed?

You may have heard the saying, "And the day came when the risk it took to remain tight in the bud became more painful than the risk it took to blossom." Or, as Tony Robbins puts it, "Change happens when the pain of staying the same is greater than the pain of change." Translated to living a life of addiction: "Change will happen for an addict (usually when they hit their bottom), when the fear and pain of remaining in the hell of being preoccupied with, imprisoned by, and powerless over food, alcohol, etc. is even less frightening than facing life without it (food, alcohol, shopping, promiscuity, internet porn, cocaine, codeine, gambling, etc.).

ABSTINENCE VS RECOVERY

Keep in mind the difference between abstinence and recovery. If you simply quit using the drug, you are "dry" (without the drug). And without the drug, you are highly vulnerable to a round at the Whack-A-Mole Addiction table.

My bottom with anorexia/food addiction came as a result of a sequence of consequences. I weighed 89 pounds, stood 5 feet, 4 inches tall, purchased clothing in the children's department, and was a sophomore in college. This disease took hold of me in a short period of time and I knew I had to get a grip or I would die.

At one point in my freshman year of college, I went "home" during a school break as I had scheduled an appointment with my dentist. During that first year of college when my daily consumption of food dwindled to a small dish of cottage cheese mixed with coleslaw, I chewed quite a bit of Grape Bubble Yum or JumBlo bubble gum balls.

All. The. Time.

I'd put an entire package of 8 pieces of Bubble Yum in my mouth at the same time. The sugar. It gave me pleasure. And it gave me energy.

It also gave me cavities. Fourteen of them in one year to be exact. Yes, I'm serious! Talk about a consequence of my addiction! Believe it or not, the dentist filled all of those suckers (sorta punny) in one visit.

Before I headed out of town to return to the isolation of

my crowded dorm, my younger brother and I hugged good-bye. He jumped back from our short hug, and nearly shrieked, "Gross! Bones!" The skin on my back was cleaving to my rib bones. I was, literally, skin and bones.

The boy I dated during my senior year of high school was attending a college a few hours drive from the big university I attended. One or the other of us would occasionally go visit the other for a weekend, although I wouldn't say we were still officially dating. On the way there, my food addiction in control, I participated in a disgusting, food-addicted behavior. I chewed up food and spit it into an empty container of some sort, one I could throw away and pretend my appalling sickness did not exist. While engaging in my chewing-for-flavor, spitting-to-avoid-calories ritual, I took my eyes off the road. When I looked up, I was in the lane for oncoming traffic. Had there been a car in that lane, I could easily have killed all involved. That would have been the lowest possible bottom. But for the grace…

The 14 cavities, my brother's horror over my boney back, and my terror of realizing I could have killed myself and/or others, got my attention. Along with one additional event.

I participated in a group on campus for females with eating disorders. The "anorexics" and the "bulimics" co-mingled for many activities, yet some interventions were disorder-specific. Given that those of us who were boney to the touch could not grasp the reality that we were not fat, one day we were instructed to bring a two-piece bathing suit to group therapy with us. The counselors took individual pictures of us in our swimsuits.

The photo of the girl they showed me was most definitely not a picture of me. *I* saw what I looked like in the mirror and the chick in that picture wearing the swimsuit (the same blue and white striped suit I had!) was not me. *I* had cellulite on my disgustingly fat thighs. *My* stomach poked out. *I* was chunky. *I* felt fat. *I* felt huge. *I* looked huge in the mirror! The child in the picture they took was emaciated and looked about ten years old! Her hipbones stuck out and so did her shoulder blades. She had no thighs and her stomach was concave. She had to be living in one of those countries they always told us had no food. She was gross. Where *had* she gotten a swimsuit that looked just like mine?

That's when I knew. I was very, very sick. What I saw and how I felt did not at all match the picture of what I looked like in reality. In reality, I looked like I was already dead.

My internal, invisible guide silently told me I needed to gain weight. But I was nowhere near ready to enter into a lifestyle of Recovery. I learned a new game instead. It was called Whack-A-Mole Addiction.

THE NEXT BIG THING

I had been working three jobs while going to school and starving myself. I walked to the Pizza Hut (oh, the irony of it all), which was a good three miles from my dorm. I'd usually get a ride home as it would be dark by the time I got off work. I was also working at a classy little bar called "The Fox Lounge," spinning records and pretending to be a D.J. (more on that momentarily). My third job was working in the dormitory cafeteria (again, around food). This job paid for my room and board, decreasing the amount of student loans I needed to take out for school.

As one may have guessed, I sucked as a DJ. I didn't talk to anyone, much less put on my Ryan Seacrest voice and get others enthused about getting out on the dance floor to shake what their mama gave 'em! I knew I sucked and so did the people who hired me. Rather than firing me, they offered to let me be a "cocktail waitress." I was underage at the time. I had turned 19 but the drinking age had been raised to 21. Somehow, I guess it was legal to serve alcohol when you were underage. I just couldn't drink it. But I did drink it! After not drinking during my freshman year (God forbid I consume liquid calories), I resumed my rabid alcohol consumption with zeal.

Resumed? Oh, I guess I hadn't mentioned that although I didn't drink frequently in high school, I drank excessively. No off switch and all that.

I honestly don't know how I didn't die of alcohol poisoning the first time I drank. It was behind my parents' back, right in front of them, at my older sister's high school graduation party. Having never touched alcohol prior to that, my 16-year-old self had no notion of how the stuff affected you. I chugged several vodka's with OJ and then my friends and I drove off to the "teen dance" at the local disco. (Who came up with such a stupid idea, anyway? Oh, wait. I know! The owners of the clubs who wanted to prep the next cohort of potential drunks!). By the time we got to the venue, I was puking and had forgotten who I was, where I was, why I was there, and who the people with me were. I remember nothing except getting sick and waking up the next day, sick as hell. I didn't drink – orange juice, that is – for a very long time after that.

Still underage while working as a cocktail waitress at the swanky Fox Lounge, I resumed my drinking career, slowly but surely. And I'll be damned if I not only started to drink again, but I resumed talking, and socializing, and dancing. And I put on weight! Alcohol, along with 2 AM trips to the local pancake house for eggs, onion rings and pancakes, put some meat on my bones and some fun into my remaining college years! (Well! I did have some fun.)

WHACK-A-MOLE ADDICTION. IN ACTION.

When a food addict has weight loss surgery, they are in serious danger of losing a game of Whack-A-Mole Addiction. This is especially true if they are not aware of food addiction, the disease. In the short time they lie sedated in the operating room, they are rendered unable to consume any solid food for quite some time. They have not entered a program of Recovery for food addiction prior to their procedure. And during the preparation for surgery and immediately following surgery, they have been thrown into abstinence, and most likely, withdrawal. At the very least, they will experience emotional withdrawal from food.

Fortunately, people are so sedated and fatigued after surgery they probably don't realize the physical withdrawal symptoms from the foods they are addicted to. It takes three to ten days for the withdrawal effects of food to stabilize. These physical withdrawal symptoms can include being shaky, nauseous, having muscle aches, and experiencing moodiness, insomnia and mental confusion.

The bariatric patient may be too physically weakened following surgery to realize that part of their misery during the recovery process may be due to withdrawal from sugar, processed flour or other foods to which they may have been addicted. However, they are often acutely aware of the psychological withdrawal.

One of my very best friends called me the day she returned home from the hospital after having the gastric sleeve procedure. Through heavy tears, she choked out, "What have I done? Why did I do this? I miss food! I MISS MY FOOD!" I had already been working in bariatrics for several years and had heard this same lament from countless patients. Working very hard to keep the chuckle threatening to escape into my telephone speaker, I comforted, "I know. It's really hard right now." I didn't have enough time to share additional sympathetic statements with her before she burst out, "No! I mean I REALLY miss food! I will **never** feel as happy as I did when I sat here on this very same couch with a huge plate of spaghetti. Maybe I'll never be happy again! Oh, God! *What have I done?*" She sobbed. I was glad at the moment that we lived in different states because I feared if I was with her I wouldn't be able to let my genuine sympathy for her sadness show through the giggles I was able to stifle hundreds of miles away.

I wasn't laughing at my friend. I know that she was dead serious about her grief. I completely sympathized with her very real loss. My silent snickers were in knowing that this would pass for her, as I had seen it do with hundreds of patients. As the weight starts to "fall off," "What have I done?" becomes "Look what I'm doing! This is the greatest thing I've ever done for myself!"

Let me be clear. There is nothing humorous about the emotional withdrawal from food. My "being tickled" by my friend's sadness was sort of like when your teenager has their wisdom teeth extracted. When you first see them after the procedure, they are doped up, groggy, and simply look tragic. They say funny things in their amnestic stupor and you just can't help but laugh and try to make it look like you're not laughing at them! You know their pain is real, and yet you know they are physically fine and will heal up nicely. That's what it was like for me with my friend after her bariatric surgery. By the way, she had called me years earlier, the day she brought her adopted son home from the hospital. Sobbing, she said to me that day, "What have I done? Oh, my God! What have I done?" He has been the light of her life every day since.

The grief of the loss of one's previous relationship with food following bariatric surgery is a very serious matter. For some people, food addict or not, food has played a significant role in their life. It was a friend, a confidant. A companion.

Food keeps many an otherwise terrifically lonely person company on yet another human-companionless night. Food, the friend, doesn't reprimand, scold or call names. It spends time with people, doesn't reject them, listens without asking questions, and asks nothing of them. On the contrary, food comforts, soothes and helps repress the too-painful reality of the loneliness.

A relationship with food can be an emotional salve, a bandage, a psychological steri-strip between the sharp edges of life's harsh realities and one's tender heart. A milkshake holds together a breaking heart like the uneven stitches that keep Raggedy Ann intact.

A head filled with rage takes out the emotion on a tub of crunchy, salty, buttery popcorn. As the contents of the bucket diminish, the greasy butter residing all over one's hands and face melt away angry emotions.

The pit in the stomach brought on by the third date in row that's been cancelled is softened and soothed by the silky smooth warmth of the chocolate squares that melt into warm bliss, coating the raw ache in the belly.

After bariatric surgery, the companion, the confidant, the painkiller referred to as food is gone. Food in these roles is lost to you. This loss can be a tremendous emotional ordeal for people who have bariatric surgery.

Losses evoke grief. Let yourself grieve. My friend was grieving when she called in her despair, wondering, "What have I done?" The unspoken question may have been, "Why did I give up my good friend? The friend I sat with on this very couch with and felt happier than I have ever felt before in my life."

Weight loss surgery requires a step-by-step reintroduction to solid foods that can last several weeks, depending on the recommendations of each program's surgeon and nutritionist. Typically, people consume a sugar-free diet that begins with clear liquids, followed by more dense liquids, then soft foods and eventually the return of solid foods. If a person carefully follows these steps in the prescribed fashion, they will have been abstinent from adding sugar to foods, (although not necessarily from refined carbohydrates).

The loss of ability to consume their favorite foods in their desired quantities causes an eruption of feelings for many post-operative patients. "I was terrified of not being able to reach for whatever food I wanted." "I went to the kitchen seven times the first evening I was home and felt lost." "I cried for a solid week." "The helplessness and hopelessness threatened to choke me." These feelings are common following weight loss surgery.

FOOD ADDICTS AFTER SURGERY

The first thing any food addict must do if they desire to live in Recovery from their addiction is to abstain from their trigger foods/substances. Food addicts who have weight loss surgery are all of a sudden abstinent from sugar and from most of the substances they turned to in the past for chemical relief. Like the loss of a job, a home, or a person, the loss of addictive foods is felt physically, emotionally and spiritually.

Grieve, my friends. Grieve the loss of food and how it "helped" you in the moment. Grieve the loss of a substance that brought you pleasure. Maybe you need to grieve the fact that there is little else in your life currently giving you pleasure. Grieve the reassurance of knowing that in your desk drawer was a never-ending supply of sugar in tidy little wrappers of bite-sized bliss. Grieve the late-night sweet indulgences that may have been the best part of your day. Grieve the simplicity of not having to think about what to cook and ease that drive-thru's provided. If food has been a friend to you, then grieve the loss of that friend.

Grieving is the beginning of the end of your unhealthy relationship with food. It is the beginning of the possibility of having a healthy relationship with food.

Weight loss surgery throws you into a ditch. Instant abstinence. For those who haven't come to terms with the fact that they have an addiction to certain foods, this will most likely be a traumatic experience! It's fairly traumatic for anyone who has weight loss surgery, regardless of whether or not they are a food addict.

If people reach out for the hands available to help them out of the ditch into which they have landed, there is hope for long-term successful weight loss. If people "do what they're told to do" after surgery, for the rest of their lives, they have a good chance of maintaining a much healthier weight than prior to having surgery. If, however, they do not "do what they're told" following surgery, many people regain some, most, or all of the weight they lost following their bariatric procedure. Some gain even more weight than they carried prior to bariatric surgery.

If you don't want to regain the weight you lose after bariatric surgery, then DO WHAT YOU'RE TOLD!

CHAPTER EIGHT

YOU'RE NOT THE BOSS OF ME

If you're a food addict, the end of the last chapter may have frustrated you: If people 'do what they're told to do' after surgery, for the rest of their lives, they have a good chance of maintaining a much healthier weight than prior to having surgery. If, however, they do not 'do what they're told' following surgery, many people regain some, most or all of their weight. Some gain even more weight than they carried prior to bariatric surgery. The simple answer, is, of course, DO WHAT YOU'RE TOLD!

I could hear frustrated voices saying, "You're not the boss of me!" Or, "Yeah, right! If you know so much about food addiction, then you oughta know there's nothing 'simple' about 'just doing what you're told.'" Pretty sure I heard some anger being sent my way, "I didn't know what food addiction was when I had bariatric surgery. How could I possibly have stuck to 'simply' doing what I was told?" "Sheesh. I thought you understood addiction. There's nothing 'simple' about it! If I could have done what I was told to do regarding food and my weight ('eat less, move more'), I wouldn't have needed bariatric surgery!"

Trust me, it was difficult for me to end that last chapter

the way I did because I DO understand addiction. I agree with the "voices" I imagined talking back to me at the close of that chapter. I work tirelessly to try to get other professionals who are involved in the world of bariatrics, whether they specialize in medical weight loss or surgical weight loss, to understand that the whole medical community is missing the boat on many counts. One day soon, I'm gonna write a book titled, Weight Loss Professionals: PULL YOUR HEADS OUT! Here are some of the points I want to highlight in that book:

- If 'eating less and moving more' were all it took for people to lose weight, then once they did those things, the problem would be solved. Clearly, there's more to this business of obesity…

- 'Behavior modification,' while essential, is not sufficient in order to help keep people doing the things they need to do in order to maintain a healthier weight… they need MORE than behavior modification techniques.

- People need to be assessed for food addiction. Traditional weight loss interventions DO NOT TREAT FOOD ADDICTION.

  - If you, Mr./Ms. Bariatric Professional do not believe in food addiction, you need to open your mind and educate yourself or receive formal education about food addiction.

  - Food addiction requires ABSTINENCE and DAILY SUPPORT.

  - Food addiction requires a daily PROGRAM of RECOVERY.

- Many people suffering from obesity, addicts and/or non-addicts, have emotional difficulties underlying their unhealthy abuse of food.

  - Depression, anxiety and other mental health issues interfere with the motivation to follow through with behavior modification. These problems need to be treated along with increased education about health and weight behaviors.

  - Shame (low self-worth, poor self-efficacy), is a central issue common to many patients struggling with

113

the disease of obesity. Continual negative self-talk reinforces low self-worth. Shame prevents people from believing in themselves enough to continue healthy behavior modifications in the long run without tremendous amounts of support.

- "Do No Harm" is the ethical code of physicians and others of us in the helping professions. By not providing patients more long-term support and treatment for food addiction when necessary, we *are* doing harm to many of our patients.

Have I reassured you that I'm not oblivious enough to believe that simply being told what to do will result in easy weight loss and maintenance? You do recall that I am in Recovery for Addictions myself, right? So no, I am well aware that there's nothing easy about recovering from an addiction. I do know it's possible. I also know that life in Recovery is beyond worth the EFFORT (a major player here) it takes to live on the colorful side of Lake Hælan.

SO PLEASE - DO WHAT YOU'RE TOLD

When I found myself in the "addict" classes at my treatment center rather than in the "family of addicts" classes, I realized the counselors there told us the exact same things to do as did the people at the various 12-Step Meetings. They said that IF we wanted to live in Recovery from our addictions, we were to do the following:

- Refrain from ALL mood-altering substances.
- Go to 12-Step Meetings regularly.
- Read the Big Book.
- Get, and utilize, a Sponsor.
- Give it away so you can keep it.

Five things. That was it. Simple. And yet, no one said it was easy. It's not easy because addicts are often afraid. Afraid of what? I know what I feared about giving up alcohol and pain medication, but I couldn't speak for other people. So I asked them on social media to, "Tell me something that an addict fears when they do not have their drug or behavior of choice available to them?" Here are some of the responses I got:

- "Being alone. There is no comfort."
- "Feeling the emotions hidden behind the food."
- "Boredom."
- "Visibility. Without all the drama and distractions of our addictions and destructive behaviors, people will see us. Vulnerability."
- "Loss of control."
- "Having nothing to dull the pain."
- "Dealing with feelings in general and shame especially."
- "It's like the loss of a best friend. What do you reach for when stressed, bored, depressed? How do I deal with the pressure of everyday life without my 'friend?'"
- "I fear loneliness and pain."
- "I seek numbness and satiety."
- "I fear failure. Of myself really. My issues with food always linger. If I let go of actively being aware in general, that's when the lingering problem becomes a reality. Then the shame and guilt can be overwhelming."
- "Going to an alternative addiction."
- "The fear of life changing. That you can never go on as before once you give up your drug."
- "Anxiety, vulnerability, fear, shame, guilt, resentment, loneliness."
- "Having to deal with the problems in my life."
- "I fear I'm not enough, like I SHOULD be able to handle things, and I become irrational. I go slightly crazy and throw temper tantrums... even if just in my mind."
- "I'm afraid of turning to something else when I need my comfort zone."
- "I fear that I will never escape this anger, that I will always feel broken. The fear gets more intense the longer I have the 'need' and can't find comfort in some way."
- "Dealing with stress."
- "I fear change itself."
- "That the demons in my head will take over."

- "That I will go nuts! It feels like that sometimes. I even dwell on what I will do in order to not give into the indulgence."
- "One word... life."
- "Feeling isolated and alone."
- "I fear the anxiety of not having what I want and the feeling of missing something so badly it makes me sad."
- "I have the fear of being able to cope."
- "Loss."
- "Being overwhelmed with emotion."
- "I fear cravings and withdrawal."
- "Losing my escape from reality."
- "Being hungry."
- "Powerlessness and rejection."
- "Not fitting in."
- "Looking stupid in situations."
- "Not knowing what to do or how to handle things in certain situations."
- "Failure."
- "Success."

Addicts were often not taught:
- Healthy expression of feelings.
- How to set healthy boundaries/how to say "No."
- Healthy communication skills (in marriage, with children & friends, etc.).
- Emotional regulation skills.
- Healthy coping skills.
- To be a healthy partner in a committed relationship.
- To be a healthy parent.
- To be a healthy friend.

After bariatric surgery, the majority of programs tell patients to:
- Follow their program's food reintroduction schedule.
- Take their vitamins as instructed.

- Engage in regular exercise.
- Attend support group meetings.
- Attend all follow-up recommended medical visits.

More comprehensive programs offer:

- Opportunities for professional counseling, if needed (some even have in-house counseling available, groups and/or individual).
- Videos to help patients better prepare for the emotional aspects related to surgery, both prior to and after surgery, as well as videos related to specific health-related topics (that would be my MindPrep series!).
- Information about... wait for it... yep! Food Addiction (although I have not seen much of this made available to patients)

One spectacular bariatric program not only offers all of the above, but also hosts a five-day retreat for all of their patients. During the retreats, patients receive information about long-term nutrition, the importance of mindfulness in eating, as well as the importance of exercise and healthy ways to deal with the stress of life. Participants engage in physical exercise and enjoy small group discussions about relationships, self-esteem, body image and food addiction. This is a comprehensive program. One I wish all bariatric programs were modeled after. It is, however, located in New Zealand.

As I mentioned in Chapter Two, most programs in the U.S. include the minimal standards of the requirements they need in order to qualify for the "Bariatric Center of Excellence" designation. While those standards cover the basics, they are sorely lacking in what patients need and want in order to deal effectively with the issues they face after bariatric surgery, one of them, for many, being food addiction.

I also mentioned there are exceptional programs here in the US doing more and more to include noteworthy pre- and post-op care for their patients. These programs and the people working for them, have my utmost respect and gratitude. I hope others take their lead.

FOOD ADDICTS: JUST DO WHAT YOU'RE TOLD TO DO

So as not to get overwhelmed, let's do as most 12-Step Recovery programs suggest and keep things simple. While I'm at it, let me clarify what I mean when I say something is simple. I am not saying the simple thing is easy. The following are *simple* tasks, meaning they are uncomplicated, plain. There is nothing complicated about being told to "Go to 12-Step Meetings." That doesn't necessarily make it an easy thing to do. One synonym for easy is "painless." Many of the meetings I have attended have been far from painless! So many of the topics discussed at 12-Step Meetings are emotionally painful. While sitting in meetings, I have heard things about addictive thinking and behavior that pertain to me and about which I feel great sadness or shame. I know when I go to a 12-Step meeting (a simple thing for me: get in my car and go to the meeting), I will likely encounter some difficult, emotionally painful topics. This makes going on a regular basis far from being easy. And yet, the gains of attending meetings far outweigh the difficulties!

Here again, is the list of things I was told to do when I was in treatment:

- Refrain from ALL mood-altering substances.
- Go to 12-Step Meetings regularly.
- Read the Big Book.
- Get, and utilize, a Sponsor.
- Give it away so you can keep it.

Here's a list of similar things for food addicts to do in order to get started in a Program of Recovery.

- Refrain from ALL mood-altering substances.
- Get, and utilize, a Sponsor.
- Go to 12-Step Meetings regularly.
- Give it away so you can keep it.
- Learn about food addiction.
- Participate in therapy.

You may have some questions about specifics related to each of these items, so I'll elaborate on them individually. You're still likely to have some questions and I certainly won't have thought of them all, so please be sure to seek answers to those questions. And remember, you have to create a program of Recovery that works for you. These are recommendations as a basis for a healthy program of recovery from food addiction to get you started on your way!

Let's get you started on your way to *doing what you're told!* And if you are the rebel of all rebels and refuse to do what you're told because someone else is telling you to do it, then figure out a way to do what they said a trillion times on American Idol and "Make it your own" idea. Because it's true, no one is the boss of you!

CHAPTER NINE

A SIMPLE PROGRAM OF RECOVERY FROM FOOD ADDICTION

Let's get on with your program of Recovery then! Oh, but before we do that, let me just say that the information in this chapter really needs to be its own book. Hey, now there's an idea! The main purpose of this book is to help you learn more about what food addiction is and to help you examine your own life to see if you have the disease of food addiction. If you have had bariatric surgery or are contemplating doing so, understanding food addiction is essential. No surgical procedure or diet will work on the addiction. You have to get treatment for addiction (food or any other) in addition to bariatric surgery in order to live your healthiest life.

What follows is a sketch of what a basis program of Recovery includes. It is not all-inclusive by any means. But it's a darn good place to get started. So without further ado, let's go!

REFRAIN FROM ALL MOOD-ALTERING SUBSTANCES (AND BEHAVIORS).

Here's the deal, and this is a hard-liner: If you want to live in

Recovery from food addiction, you literally cannot have your cake and eat it, too. And it's not just the cake you can't have. It's whatever foods and food substances "trigger you." Those two words, "trigger you," probably don't need explanation. If you are clueless about what people mean when they say something like, "I don't eat _____ because it 'triggers me,'" then I'm guessing you're not a food addict, although I've been wrong before! ☺

When a food addict is "triggered" by a specific food or food substance, they say things like this:

- "From the first bite of _____, I'm hooked and can't think of anything else."

- "It's off to the sugar races for me if I so much as eat one chocolate kiss."

- "I hope when I die there's a mashed potato heaven because mashed potatoes are too dangerous for me to have the first bite in my human form."

- "Once I get started, I'll eat everything in the house that contains sugar."

- "Once I give in to sweets, it is truly like living in an altered state of mind. My thinking is foggy, my body is sluggish, and I simply crave and crave anything sweet."

- "A thousand cookies is not enough and one is too many."

- "I have to stay away from carbs or I'll eat them until I feel sick."

IF YOU CAN'T "TAKE IT OR LEAVE IT," OR IF "FOOD CALLS" TO YOU, THEN ALL FOODS THAT TRIGGER YOU OR LEAVE YOU CRAVING MORE AND MORE, ARE OFF LIMITS.

If you've done much reading about food addiction, then you know that sugar, flour, wheat, refined foods, oily and starchy foods, and the combination of these foods are the most common food trigger substances. For some people, artificial sweeteners also result in excessive use and/or cravings.

START A LIST OF FOODS THAT ARE OFF LIMITS FOR YOU. ADD TO IT AS NEEDED.

Start a list of foods that trigger you. Continue to add foods as you realize they render you "helpless" for wanting more, leave you obsessing about food, or trigger you to get more of that food or similar foods.

How many people are actually willing to make a list of foods from which they choose to remain abstinent? I don't know, but I've only met a few myself. For many a reason, people don't want to let 'their' cookies or 'their' ice cream or 'their' particular food go. Continuing to eat foods you are addicted to makes being in Recovery impossible.

FOR ADDICTS, ABSTINENCE IS ESSENTIAL FOR RECOVERY.

Have you ever noticed how people with addictions often take personal ownership of food, alcohol, or other substances?

"What? Give up my sweet tea? I'd rather lose all my teeth."

"I have to have my mint chip before bed."

"I'm gonna have my beer at night and my cocktails on the weekend."

"I'd give up social media or television before I'd give up my pain meds. I gotta have those."

It's like Linus from Charlie Brown. He always has his security blankie. Or like the two-year-old with only a few words to her vocabulary. She definitely knows the words, "MY paci." Yes, noting the infantile comfort items is intentional. I often find myself giggling, thinking of a room filled with adults, imagining the addicts in the room with pacifiers made to resemble their addictive substance of choice hanging out of their mouths. Can you picture it:

- the attorney with a plastic pacifier in the shape of a martini glass?
- the prim and proper schoolteacher whose paci looks like a piece of lemon meringue pie?
- the bus driver with a blunt-shaped pacifier?
- the surgeon whose paci resembles a prescription bottle holding the equivalent of speed to help him stay awake?
- the minister with a pacifier that looks like a computer screen representing internet pornography? (it happens a lot, I'm afraid)
- the administrative assistant with a pacifier resembling Mt.

Rushmore, depicting the number of men she's currently sleeping with?

- the food addiction therapist whose pacifier looks like the puke bag on an airplane, indicating her own struggle with bulimia?

There would be so many more "pacis" in that room than you would imagine. There are a lot of "functional addicts" in any crowd. In any room with adults, addictions are alive and well. We're human. Many of us were never taught healthy coping skills to deal with stress. A lot of us were raised in chaotic homes. Very many of us have genetic predispositions to addiction.

Most people battling addictions are caught in the web of denial about them. Of those that are aware, few have the knowledge, wisdom or courage about how to deal head-on with their addictions.

Addiction is real. Food addiction is real. Some people are physically triggered by foods. Others have emotional addictions to food. The idea of giving them up is terrifying. What will they do when they are upset with their boss, spouse, child or parent and don't have food for comfort? How will they get through a lonely, friendless weekend if they don't have their usual edible companions? What will they turn to when they can't keep their anger in, and only the cooling effects of a milkshake have proven to decrease their rage?

Following weight loss surgery, a person needs to continue identifying foods that have been, or become, off-limits. Nicky did remarkably well after her gastric bypass. She lost 137 pounds in 11 months following her procedure. She hired a personal trainer and was working out with a group of friends four times a week. Her business was flourishing and her marriage improving. Nicky continued to see me on a monthly basis to "stay grounded." One day, about 20 months after she had surgery, continuing to maintain her weight loss, Nicky told me she had a "confession" to make. Several months prior she had taken up the habit of having a prune with peanut butter as a mid-afternoon snack. The prune helped keep her "regular," and the natural peanut butter was a reasonable source of fat and protein. The "confession" was that her afternoon snack of prunes and peanut butter had increased to 8 prunes covered with peanut butter in one sitting. This combination was wreaking havoc in her life, as you can imagine. In addition to being "regular" all day long, she was consuming an enormous number of calories in her "afternoon snack." Prunes, and peanut butter went on her list of trigger foods that she no longer ate.

Any food can end up on your list, depending on how honest you are willing to be.

OTHER MOOD-ALTERING SUBSTANCES AND BEHAVIORS

But wait, there's more! I don't want anyone playing a losing game of Whack-A-Mole Addiction. Remember, most addicts don't engage in just one form of addiction. Some participate in multiple addictions at the same time. Others seem to flow from one destructive addiction to another, usually adopting a new one when some other is given up.

Mood-altering substances include alcohol, narcotics (prescribed or otherwise), cigarettes, caffeine, and all street drugs, "legalized" or not. Mood-altering behaviors can include excess: shopping, social networking, cleaning, reading, gambling, sex, internet pornography, or online sexting. Any behavior done in excess that interferes in your life is a problem. If something is creating problems, then it's a problem.

I'm not telling you not to have a cup of coffee. If you have excessive coffee to the point you're so jittery you can't do you work, you should probably cut way back or quit. If coffee leads to an irregular heartbeat and your doctor has told you to stop and you don't, then I'd call that a problem.

I'm certainly not saying don't read a book to relax, to learn or to laugh. If you're reading so much that your children can't get your attention when they need you, that's probably using reading in a problematic manner.

Be honest with yourself. Listen to people who have expressed concern about your use of alcohol or drugs, excessive cleaning or talking on the phone to the point of neglecting your work or family. Be extremely careful not to increase the use of mood-altering substances or behaviors of any kind as you begin your process of Recovery.

It is likely that over time, not only will you add more and more foods to your list of that you choose to abstain from, but you will also recognize, and eliminate other unhealthy behaviors. Like cigarettes, if you're a smoker. There's no way around it. Cigarettes are deadly. I wasn't willing to give them up at the time I quit drinking and threw away the narcotic medication I was addicted to. In fact, I had quit smoking previously and started smoking again when I was in treatment. I did quit within a year. But please quit smoking. Please. And if prunes and peanut butter become an issue for you, well… you know what to do!

YES, IT'S HARD

Giving up specific foods, food groups, and other mood-altering substances and behaviors is exceptionally difficult for most people. That's why living a solid, healthy program of Recovery provides additional guidelines which offer the support you need to live free from your "foods (drug) of choice":

- Get, and utilize, a Sponsor.
- Go to 12-Step Meetings regularly.
- Learn about food addiction.
- Give it away so you can keep it.
- Participate in therapy.

GET, AND UTILIZE, A SPONSOR.

A sponsor. A sponsor is someone who will support you as you do the work, and I do mean WORK, required to live in Recovery from your addiction(s). Remember the list of fears people shared in relation to giving up their addiction? You have to work hard learning and following healthy options for dealing with those fears to remain sober and in Recovery. Believe it or not, fears and not knowing how to cope with them in healthy ways often lead to relapse. Support is essential, as you learn to face the stressful, fearful realities of life without mood-altering addictions.

Bariatric centers do provide options for support following bariatric surgery. Patients have some access (hopefully) to the staff at their bariatric center. Support groups, typically offered once a month, provide some support. Online bariatric groups, some affiliated with a bariatric program, also provide support. These are good options, without a doubt! But none take the place of a sponsor.

A sponsor in a program of Recovery, is someone who has been down the road before you, has experienced the bumps in the road, has fallen in the potholes, and has survived the unforeseen twists and turns. They may have landed in a ditch a time or two along their own journey. They know the need for help from others in order to climb out of ditches. A sponsor understands the importance of extending a hand

and asking for assistance to get back on the road.

A good sponsor will set healthy boundaries with you. They will give you "assignments" previously given to them by their sponsors and supporters. The homework is designed to help you get to know yourself better by evaluating your thoughts and your behavior. Your sponsor will expect you to be in touch with them, and will meet with you regularly. They will hug you when you need a hug, they will listen to you, they will talk to you, and they will give you a loving kick in the arse when need be.

Your sponsor cannot be there for you at ALL times, but they *are* there for you. They will get back to you. They care about you. They will introduce you to others who will care about, and help you in Recovery. It is with the help of your sponsor and the others in the program that you will learn healthy coping skills, healthy communication skills, how to set boundaries with others, and how to better care for yourself. They help you learn to live without your drug, the foods you need to abstain from.

A sponsor will help you learn tips for getting through cravings, encourage you to deal with your fears, and will share their success stories and those of others who are working a healthy program of Recovery. Sponsors work through the twelve steps with you if you choose to participate in a 12-Step program. They will hold your feet to the fire when you engage in the "isms" of addiction. They've been there. They know the ropes. They are willing to be with you on your journey. But they cannot do the work for you. Only you can do that.

No one can do it for you. Only you can admit you're an addict. Only you can seek help. Only you can forego trigger foods and other mood-altering substances and behaviors. But you can't do a program of Recovery alone. So do this next thing.

GO TO 12-STEP MEETINGS REGULARLY

Yes, there are many roads to Rome, so if you are absolutely opposed to the 12-Step meetings, by all means, find another road! I happen to like the 12-Step programs, but am aware that they are not the be all and end all for all. By 12-Step programs, I am referring to Alcoholic Anonymous (AA), Overeaters Anonymous (OA), FA (Food Addicts in Recovery), FAA (Food Addicts Anonymous), and SAA (Sex Addicts Anonymous). There are many others. Celebrate Recovery is also a very good program. And I'm certain there are others.

The point is, you're going to need support. A lot of support. Those who have shared similar experiences will be your greatest source of support. In the book, Food Junkies by Vera Tarman and Philip Werdell, the authors share many examples of food addicts who attended AA meetings because there were no other 12-Step meetings available where they lived. By substituting "food" when they heard people talk about alcohol, the food addicts were able to learn healthy coping skills for life and learn tips for successfully working through cravings. Anyone in a program of Recovery from addiction can be a help to another addict, regardless of the specific addiction.

The majority of people present at Recovery meetings, 12-Step or other types, want what you want: relief from their addictive behaviors and information on healthier ways to cope with life. They are struggling in many of the same ways you are. They have similar histories and similar battles. I have never been to a 12-Step meeting where I did not take away something positive that helped me in my daily life.

I have, however, been to meetings where a whole lot of unhealthy behavior takes place. Beware of "13th Steppers," who are people looking to "hook up" (yes, in a sexual way). It appears Whack-A-Mole Addiction is active even at 12-Step meetings! There are also meetings with "cliques" who monopolize or leave others out. Remember, most of us start these programs with a lot of underlying "issues" that render our behavior unhealthy in ways that reach beyond our addictive actions.

"Stick with the winners" is another wonderful recovery slogan. Associate with people who look and sound like they are "walking the walk" and not just "talking the talk." Avoid people who are gossiping about others in the group. Steer clear of people who regularly bitch and moan and sound like Eeyore. Move toward those who are working a solid program of Recovery, which shows in their actions and their words. Remember, Recovery is about "progress, not perfection." No one at any meeting will be living or working a perfect program of Recovery. Nor will you or I. Ever. But put forth effort every single day to make progress.

The people at the Recovery meetings will be essential for your ongoing sobriety. You will get the phone numbers of people you can call any time you are having a "moment." These people, regardless of how well you know them, are there for you. If they have shared their telephone number with you, then they have invited you contact them. When you are having a craving, if you are feeling overwhelmed, when your partner frustrates you, when your boss upsets you, when your children annoy you, rather than turning to food, continue to call people from meetings until someone answers. Then talk it through. This works. No one can make the decision for you about whether you put food in your mouth except for you. However, the decision to refrain is much easier when you turn to others for help. Do it. The people in the Recovery programs are there to help you. They can educate you. But you need to take responsibility for learning more about addiction and Recovery on your own time.

LEARN ABOUT FOOD ADDICTION

Learn not only about food addiction, but about addiction in general. It should be clear to you by now that few people struggle with only one addiction. Some people engage in several addictions simultaneously, while others move from one to the next to the next. Learn about Recovery. Immerse yourself in this learning. Learn about the biology of addiction. Learn about the "isms" I mentioned. Become informed about the various Recovery philosophies and programs available. Find one that fits your needs and your personality. Discover what areas of life your addiction has affected (you'll be amazed). Investigate your family history. You may be surprised to learn there is much more addiction in your ancestry than you realized.

The complexity of addiction and Recovery cannot be portrayed in these few chapters. If "Addiction" and "Recovery" were to post their relationship status on social media, it would be "COMPLICATED." Addiction has, as Dr. Gabor Maté, a psychiatrist whose work in addiction is renowned, states addiction has "biological, chemical, neurological, psychological, medical, emotional, social, political, economic, and spiritual underpinnings—and perhaps others I haven't thought about." (You can watch many free talks by Dr. Maté on YouTube. I highly recommend that you do.)

To gain an understanding of food addiction from a medical perspective, read Food Junkies by Dr. Vera Tarman and Philip Werdell, which has been mentioned several times in this book. This is the best book I've read for providing an understandable medical explanation about addiction. The fact that Dr. Tarman is herself a recovering food addict adds to her knowledge of how to best treat food addiction.

Another of my favorites on the topic is <u>Shades of Hope: How to Treat Your Addiction to Food</u> by Tennie McCarty. She delineates many helpful exercises you can complete on your own throughout the book.

Immerse yourself in the knowledge of how to live a healthy life in Recovery from addiction. Read and listen from a variety of sources. The process of Recovery is, at times, emotionally painful. There are periods of time when the process is more difficult than others. It is imperative to have the tools you learn in a Recovery program at your fingertips, on your smart phone, emblazoned in your memory and tattooed on your skin if that helps! Recovery as a way of life is a mindset, a way of thinking. You are new to this way of living and thinking. Hence, the need to be inundated with information and surrounded by people who understand what you are going through.

"Back in the day," as they say, when I entered treatment and began my program of Recovery, we listened to cassette tape recordings of circuit AA speakers. I listened to numerous recordings of people who had been clean and sober for decades. These people shared their "experience, strength and hope" so that others could learn from them how to live healthy lives without using addictive substances or engaging in addictive behaviors. That is the reason people in Recovery say, "You have to give it away so you can keep it." By sharing what you have been through, you are helping others, and also reinforcing your own Recovery.

In addition to listening to recordings, I read books about people's personal stories of living in the turmoil of addiction and their transition into living joyful lives in Recovery. There were several movies that came out "on the big screen" during those years, as well. <u>Clean and Sober</u> with Michael Keaton, <u>Requiem for a Dream</u>, <u>When a Man Loves a Woman</u> with Meg Ryan, and <u>28 Days</u> with Sandra Bullock. Every day I read my daily readings from Recovery books published by Hazelden. I still do, although now they are downloaded onto my cell phone.

I went to 12-Step meetings, at least three a week in the first several years. Steve and I started spending time with couples our age also in Recovery. Our kids played together and our families enjoyed life focused on Recovery principles.

We immersed ourselves in learning about, and living a life of Recovery. That is what it takes to retrain your brain to think healthier thoughts, to learn coping skills that will serve you well, and to realize there is a good life available to you, free from the burden of addiction.

And of course, there was therapy. Lots of therapy.

GIVE IT AWAY SO YOU CAN KEEP IT.

Word-of-mouth advertising is one of the best forms of advertising any merchant can hope for! In the matter of living in Recovery from food addiction, you know you're not alone in your struggles. By sharing what you learn with others who are addressing similar issues, you both benefit! If you listen to a great podcast, whether it addresses healthy self-esteem, ways to set boundaries, positive self-talk, healthy communication skills or is more specifically oriented toward Recovery from food addiction, suggest that others listen to it! If you read a blog that helps you with cravings, let others know. If an online video assists you in learning to eat mindfully, recommend others watch it. Giving away information you have come across, not only points another person in a healthy direction, it reminds you of what you are learning!

THERAPY.

Again, I admit my bias in this area. I believe therapy is extremely important for people struggling with addictions. Although it is true that some people who are addicted to food can go about living healthy physical and emotional lives once they refrain from engaging in the foods that cause them problems, many more people need the assistance of a full program of recovery, as well as therapy.

In therapy, unlike at 12-Step meetings, you are afforded the opportunity to "clean out your emotional closet," as I refer to the process of dealing with lingering emotional baggage. Therapy helps you bridge your present life with your past. This is important in order to make connections between things that happened earlier in your life and your present behavior. This process also allows you better insight into how to make positive changes in your present life so as to have a better future. I'm not all about reviewing every detail of your history. However, I do find it useful to put pieces together, to learn from history and decide how you want to live in the present. I also believe people can make positive changes without addressing the "why" behind each and every aspect of their life. Therapy moves in a lot of different directions, depending on what your individual needs are.

From a personal standpoint, I know that therapy was

tremendously helpful for me, for Steve, for our marriage and for our family. When we were with the right therapist. The connection you have with a therapist is truly therapeutic in and of itself. Recall my intuitive sense that the young woman I first had as a therapist at the Community Mental Health Center was not a good fit for me. I had another therapist immediately after I went through treatment in the "Aftercare" portion of my process. I knew that she was the wrong therapist for me. After working hard to "keep coming back," I trusted my instincts where this woman was concerned. I didn't quit therapy. Instead, I found the therapist who has been one of the most influential people in my entire life.

Karen was the epitome of "firm and fair," which is how I refer to my therapy style. She was no-nonsense, give-it-to-you-straight, and very kind and trustworthy at the same time. I needed someone who wasn't going to baby me, who would hold my feet to the fire, all the while having my best interests at heart. Karen believed in me when I didn't believe in myself. She never babied me, but always nurtured me. She helped me grow into a much better me, guiding me, not telling me what to do. She allowed me to figure things out on my own, but was willing to give me clues along the way. She educated me in so many ways about life and people and myself. She didn't do any of the work I needed to do in order to make the changes in my life, yet her presence, her insights, and her caring made a lot of difference in my following through with positive behaviors.

In therapy, we learned a lot of things 12-Step meetings are not meant to deal with directly. Steve and I were able to practice communication exercises in our couple's therapy. By observing other couples participate in exercises in group couple's therapy, each couple learned from the others about what healthy marriages are supposed to be like. In our family therapy sessions, we learned about healthier ways to parent our children and how to work together as we raised our babies. Steve had his issues to address in his individual therapy and I got the opportunity to address mine in my individual therapy.

We were barely scraping by financially at that time in our lives and our insurance didn't cover therapy. Together we made the decision that our lives, our marriage, and our family were worth whatever the financial cost was. We paid those therapy bills for years, and are grateful for the gifts we gave ourselves by doing so.

Personally, I got so much out of therapy that I went back to school for another seven years to become a therapist! And believe me, I didn't like school the first 16 years I was in it. I had no intention of ever returning to a program of formal education. Until I started my Master's degree, four years after beginning my journey into Recovery from addiction. I haven't been able to get enough information and education about addiction and recovery and the workings of human beings since.

Give yourself the gift of therapy. Be sure you find a therapist you're comfortable with. One you trust. When you do, encourage yourself to step out of your comfort zone and talk about things that may be a bit difficult to discuss. Be open to feedback. And between sessions, give time and a lot of thought to the things you are dealing with in your sessions. Use the opportunity to let therapy help you become the best you possible.

TAKE WHAT YOU LIKE...

As they say in recovery circles, "Take what you like and leave the rest." The information in this book is offered as part of what you embrace to live a life in Recovery from addiction. Take the pieces that fit best for who you are and add them to the repertoire of skills that already works for you. If certain things I've said just don't "fit" for you, then they don't fit. They may another day or another year, but they may also never "fit" for you.

Your program of Recovery will include things you learn from a variety of sources. DO take what you like. And keep it. And use it. Live in Recovery from food addiction (and all addictions) for the rest of your life, a day at a time. Live free in Recovery from whatever ails you. Recovery from... I mean, FOR Life! Watch for that title. Coming in the not-too-distant future!

Until then, my yoga-practicing self says to you, "NAMASTE," the good in you being acknowledged by the good in me. Being in Recovery from addiction can bring out the best in us all. Here's to our best!